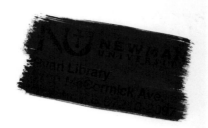

THE
VISIBLE
HUMAN
BODY

AN ATLAS OF SECTIONAL ANATOMY

GUNTHER VON HAGENS

Dr. Med.
Doctor of Medicine
Institute for Anatomy and Cell Biology
University of Heidelberg
Heidelberg, West Germany

Lynn J. Romrell

Ph.D.
Professor
Department of Anatomy and Cell Biology
University of Florida School of Medicine
Gainesville, Florida

Michael H. Ross

Ph.D.
Professor and Chairman
Department of Anatomy and Cell Biology
University of Florida School of Medicine
Gainesville, Florida

Klaus Tiedemann

Prof. Dr. Med. Vet.
Institute for Anatomy and Cell Biology
University of Heidelberg
Heidelberg, West Germany

THE VISIBLE HUMAN BODY

AN ATLAS OF SECTIONAL ANATOMY

LEA & FEBIGER, Philadelphia, London 1991

Lea & Febiger
200 Chester Field Parkway
Malvern, Pennsylvania 19355
U.S.A
(215) 251-2230
1-800-444-1785

Lea & Febiger (UK) Ltd.
145a Croydon Road
Beckenham, Kent BR3 3RB
U.K.

Reprints of chapters may be purchased from Lea & Febiger in quantities of 100 or more.

Library of Congress Cataloging-in-Publication Data

The Visible human body: an atlas of sectional anatomy/Gunther von Hagens...[et al.].
    p.   cm.
    ISBN 0-8121-1269-5
    1. Human anatomy—Atlases.   I. Hagens, Gunther von.
    [DNLM: 1. Anatomy, Regional—atlases.   QS 17 V831]
QM25.V56 1990
611' .0022'2—dc20
DNLM/DLC
for Library of Congress
                          89-13836
                                CIP

PRINTED IN SINGAPORE

Print number: 5   4   3   2   1

PREFACE

This atlas of sectional anatomy follows many others that have appeared during recent years. The impetus for most of these works, that is, the depiction of the human body viewed in slices, is related to several of the new technologies that now exist in clinical medicine. We are referring, of course, to techniques such as ultrasonography, computed tomography (CT), and magnetic resonance imaging (MRI). These new imaging techniques require that the medical student, as well as the physician and the specialized medical technologist working in this field, understand the structural relationships of the body from a perspective different from that observed during dissection of a cadaver or conventional radiography. Medical students, residents, and practitioners of radiography, surgery, and medicine must develop a concept of the body in three-dimensions and must be able to recognize structures viewed in various planes.

To improve on the currently available teaching materials for sectional anatomy, we chose to produce an atlas of color photographs of plastinated specimens. In the plastination technique, the body is sliced in the frozen state at a thickness of 2.5 to 4 mm. The sections are processed to remove water and lipids and replace them with cured epoxy polymers. The clearing of fat tissue without destruction of the connective tissue stroma, combined with the thinness of the section, results in enhanced contrast and sharper definition of structure. Moreover, structural relations are exceedingly well retained. The advantages of the sheet plastination technique are apparent in the photographs that follow.*

The students in our Gross Anatomy courses at the University of Heidelberg and at the University of Florida are enthusiastic about the use of these specimens; correlating structures in the dissected cadaver with these sections creates a more vivid and understandable mental image of three-dimensional relationships. The study of the plastinated specimens also facilitates the interpretation of radiographic, MR, and CT images. Similarly, we hope that the photographs of the specimens included in this atlas enable the user to better visualize the body utilizing modern imaging modalities, whether that individual be a student of gross anatomy, a practicing physician, or a health care specialist seeking a basic understanding of sectional anatomy.

Heidelberg	G. von Hagens
Gainesville	L.J. Romrell
Gainesville	M.H. Ross
Heidelberg	K. Tiedemann

*The plastination technique has recently been reviewed. See von Hagens, G., Tiedemann, K., and Kriz, W.: The current potential of plastination. Anat. Embrol., 175: 411-421, 1987.

ACKNOWLEDGMENTS

The authors are indebted to Mr. Achim Heckert of Heidenheim, W. Germany, for photographing the plastinated sections. His expertise enable us to obtain positive transparencies that yielded maximal detail of structure. We are equally grateful to Mr. Rudolf Partsch, of Heidenheim, for his assistance and critical involvement in the project. We also wish to express our appreciation to Ms. Regina Cheong for the line drawings she created to depict the cut represented by each of the plastinated specimens.

Special recognition is extended to Thurman Gillespy, III, M.D., of the Department of Radiology, University of Florida College of Medicine, for his assistance in the selection of CTs and MRIs included in the Atlas. We especially appreciate the considerable time that Dr. Gillespy devoted to this project in providing advice and guidance with respect to identifying the clinically important CT and MRI images. In the same vein we wish to thank Edward V. Staab, M.D., Chairman of the Department of Radiology, for his assistance and interest in the project.

Lastly, we acknowledge the advice and assistance provided by the staff of Lea & Febiger; special thanks are due to Mr. Samuel A. Rondinelli and Mr. Robert Spahr for their direct and valued participation throughout the course of this project.

CONTENTS

Part I

Head and Neck

Plates 1-1 to 1-31

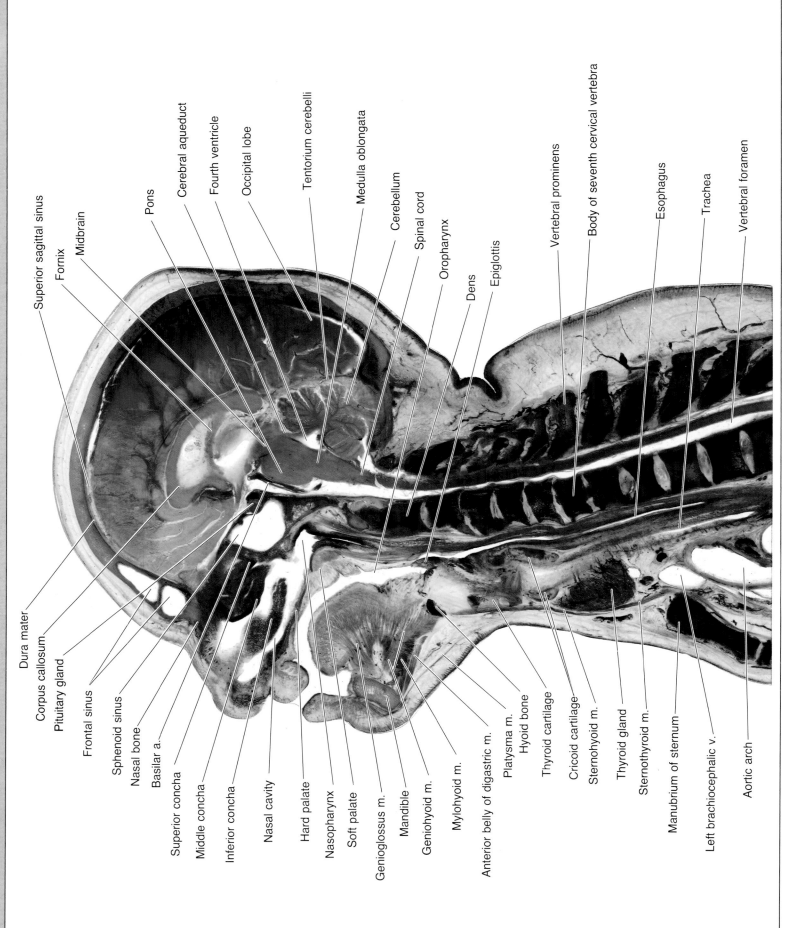

Dura mater
Corpus callosum
Pituitary gland
Frontal sinus
Sphenoid sinus
Nasal bone
Basilar a.
Superior concha
Middle concha
Inferior concha
Nasal cavity
Hard palate
Nasopharynx
Soft palate
Genioglossus m.
Mandible
Geniohyoid m.
Mylohyoid m.
Anterior belly of digastric m.
Platysma m.
Hyoid bone
Thyroid cartilage
Cricoid cartilage
Sternohyoid m.
Thyroid gland
Sternothyroid m.
Manubrium of sternum
Left brachiocephalic v.
Aortic arch

Superior sagittal sinus
Fornix
Midbrain
Pons
Cerebral aqueduct
Fourth ventricle
Occipital lobe
Tentorium cerebelli
Medulla oblongata
Cerebellum
Spinal cord
Oropharynx
Dens
Epiglottis
Vertebral prominens
Body of seventh cervical vertebra
Esophagus
Trachea
Vertebral foramen

HEAD AND NECK
Plate 1 – 1

Sagittal Section

The plane of section passes slightly to the right of the median plane exposing the concha in the
nasal cavity and passes through the frontal and sphenoid sinuses.

THE VISIBLE HUMAN BODY

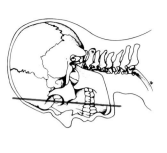

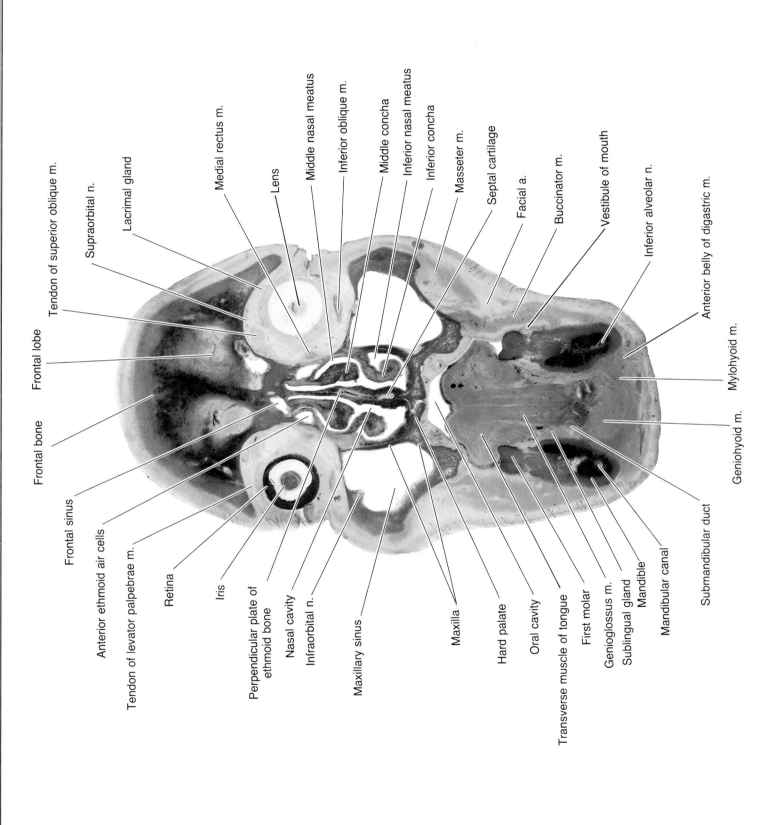

Frontal lobe

Tendon of superior oblique m.

Supraorbital n.

Lacrimal gland

Medial rectus m.

Lens

Middle nasal meatus

Inferior oblique m.

Middle concha

Inferior nasal meatus

Inferior concha

Masseter m.

Septal cartilage

Facial a.

Buccinator m.

Vestibule of mouth

Inferior alveolar n.

Anterior belly of digastric m.

Mylohyoid m.

Geniohyoid m.

Submandibular duct

Mandibular canal

Mandible

Sublingual gland

Genioglossus m.

First molar

Transverse muscle of tongue

Oral cavity

Hard palate

Maxilla

Maxillary sinus

Infraorbital n.

Nasal cavity

Perpendicular plate of ethmoid bone

Iris

Retina

Tendon of levator palpebrae m.

Anterior ethmoid air cells

Frontal sinus

Frontal bone

Coronal Section

The plane of section passes through the anterior portion of the orbits and the nasal cavity. The frontal and maxillary sinuses are included in the section.

HEAD AND NECK
Plate 1 – 2

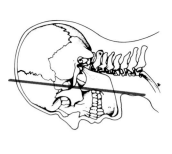

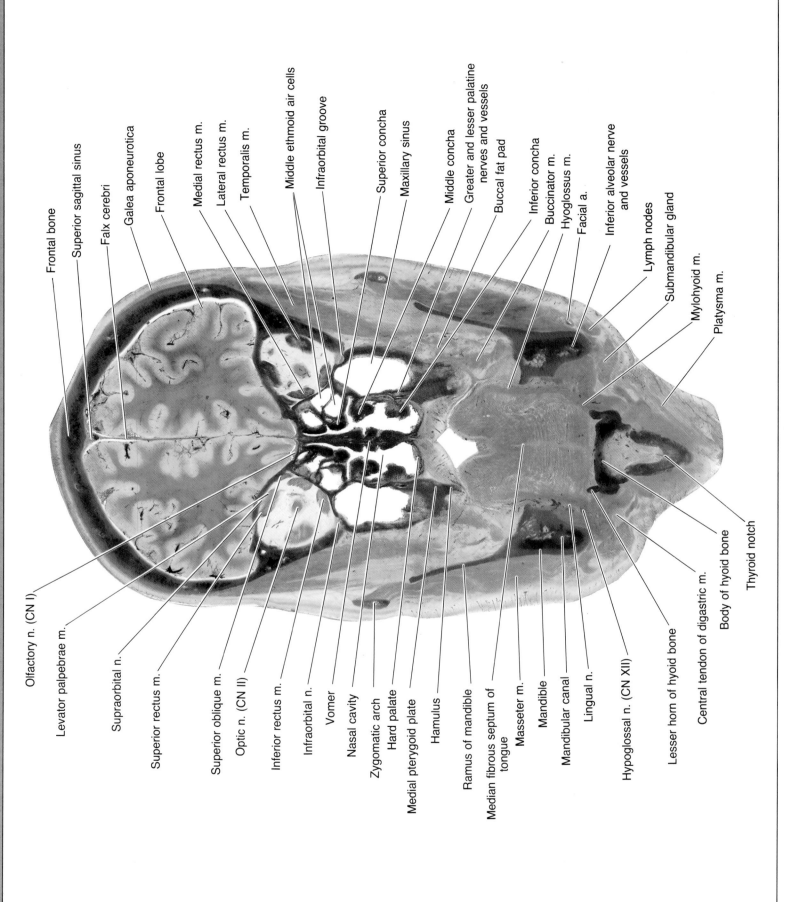

Olfactory n. (CN I)

Levator palpebrae m.

Supraorbital n.

Superior rectus m.

Superior oblique m.

Optic n. (CN II)

Inferior rectus m.

Infraorbital n.

Vomer

Nasal cavity

Zygomatic arch

Hard palate

Medial pterygoid plate

Hamulus

Ramus of mandible

Median fibrous septum of tongue

Masseter m.

Mandible

Mandibular canal

Lingual n.

Hypoglossal n. (CN XII)

Lesser horn of hyoid bone

Central tendon of digastric m.

Body of hyoid bone

Thyroid notch

Frontal bone

Superior sagittal sinus

Falx cerebri

Galea aponeurotica

Frontal lobe

Medial rectus m.

Lateral rectus m.

Temporalis m.

Middle ethmoid air cells

Infraorbital groove

Superior concha

Maxillary sinus

Middle concha

Greater and lesser palatine nerves and vessels

Buccal fat pad

Inferior concha

Buccinator m.

Hyoglossus m.

Facial a.

Inferior alveolar nerve and vessels

Lymph nodes

Submandibular gland

Mylohyoid m.

Platysma m.

The plane of section passes through the posterior portion of the orbit and the nasal cavity.
Middle ethmoid air cells and the maxillary sinus are included in the section.

Coronal Section

HEAD AND NECK
Plate 1 – 3

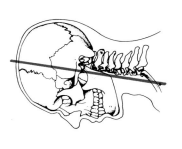

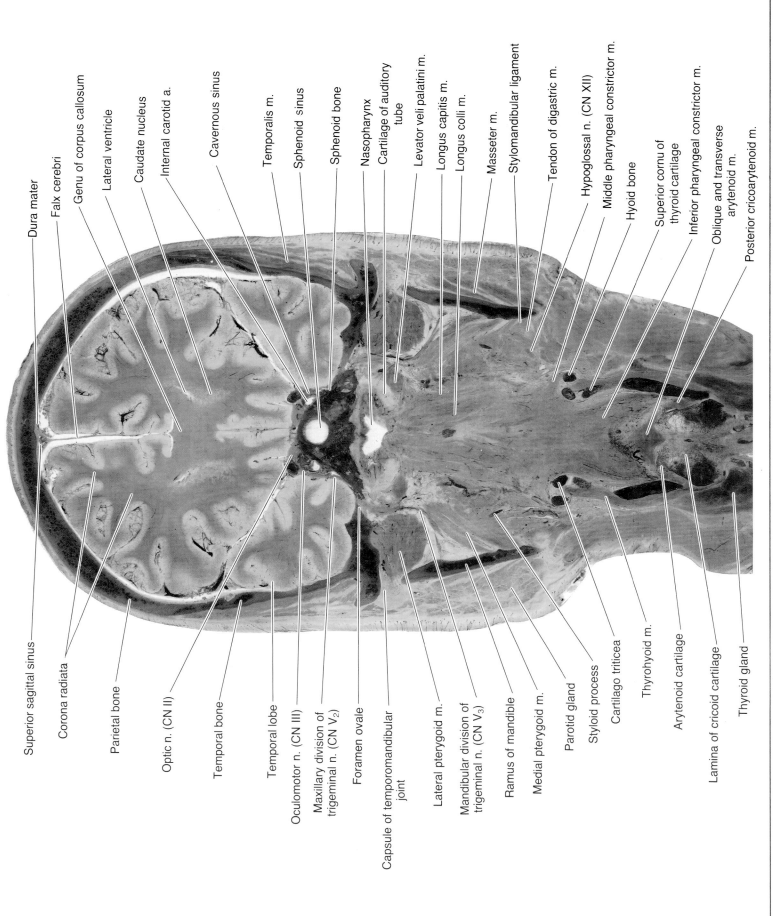

Superior sagittal sinus

Dura mater

Falx cerebri

Corona radiata

Genu of corpus callosum

Parietal bone

Lateral ventricle

Caudate nucleus

Internal carotid a.

Optic n. (CN II)

Cavernous sinus

Oculomotor n. (CN III)

Temporal bone

Maxillary division of
trigeminal n. (CN V₂)

Temporalis m.

Temporal lobe

Sphenoid sinus

Sphenoid bone

Foramen ovale

Nasopharynx

Cartilage of auditory
tube

Capsule of temporomandibular
joint

Levator veli palatini m.

Longus capitis m.

Lateral pterygoid m.

Longus colli m.

Mandibular division of
trigeminal n. (CN V₃)

Masseter m.

Stylomandibular ligament

Ramus of mandible

Tendon of digastric m.

Medial pterygoid m.

Hypoglossal n. (CN XII)

Parotid gland

Middle pharyngeal constrictor m.

Styloid process

Hyoid bone

Cartilago triticea

Superior cornu of
thyroid cartilage

Thyrohyoid m.

Inferior pharyngeal constrictor m.

Arytenoid cartilage

Oblique and transverse
arytenoid m.

Lamina of cricoid cartilage

Posterior cricoarytenoid m.

Thyroid gland

The plane of section passes through the sphenoid sinus and includes portions of the nasopharynx and larynx.
It includes the mandibular nerve as it passes through the foramen ovale.

Coronal Section

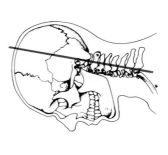

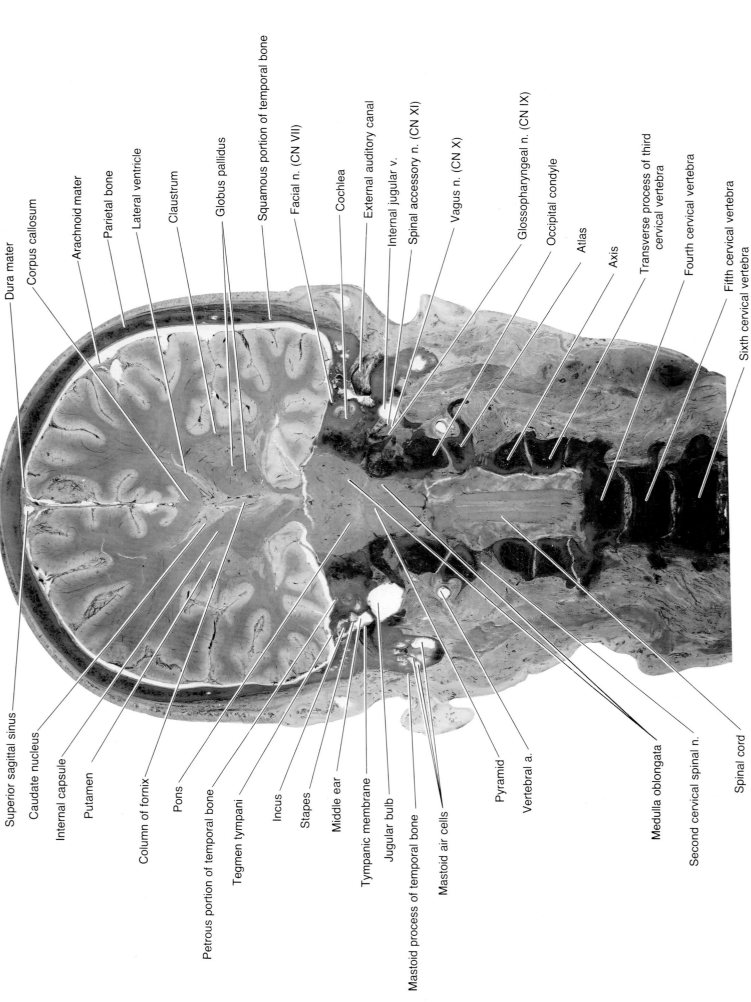

Superior sagittal sinus
Caudate nucleus
Internal capsule
Putamen
Column of fornix
Pons
Petrous portion of temporal bone
Tegmen tympani
Incus
Stapes
Middle ear
Tympanic membrane
Jugular bulb
Mastoid process of temporal bone
Mastoid air cells
Pyramid
Vertebral a.
Medulla oblongata
Second cervical spinal n.
Spinal cord

Dura mater
Corpus callosum
Arachnoid mater
Parietal bone
Lateral ventricle
Claustrum
Globus pallidus
Squamous portion of temporal bone
Facial n. (CN VII)
Cochlea
External auditory canal
Internal jugular v.
Spinal accessory n. (CN XI)
Vagus n. (CN X)
Glossopharyngeal n. (CN IX)
Occipital condyle
Atlas
Axis
Transverse process of third cervical vertebra
Fourth cervical vertebra
Fifth cervical vertebra
Sixth cervical vertebra

Coronal Section

The plane of section passes through the petrous portion of the temporal bone and includes portions of the middle and inner ear. Portions of the brain stem and spinal cord are included in the section.

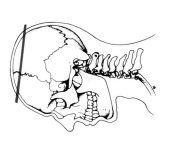

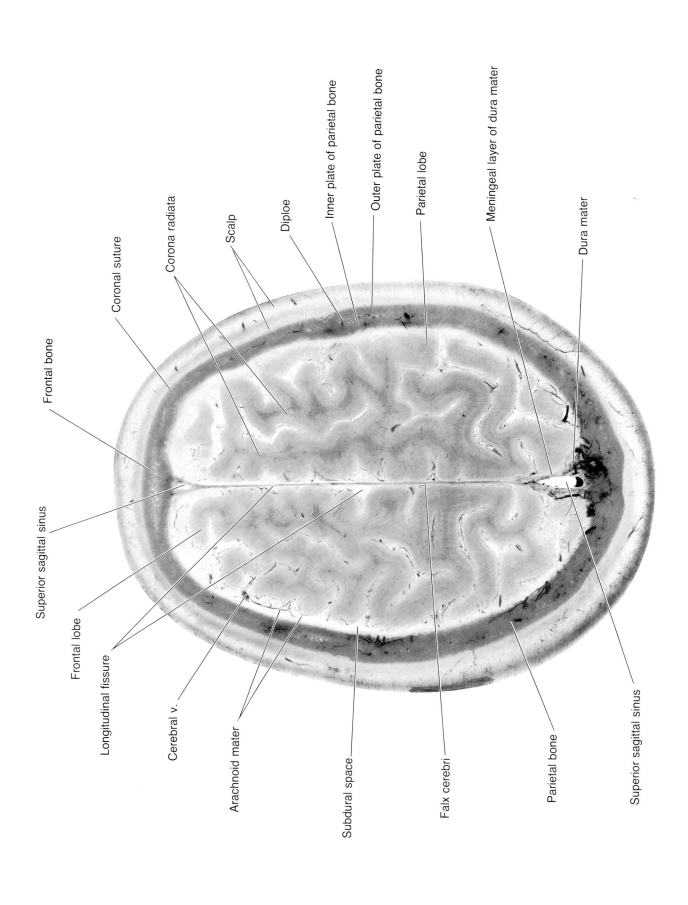

Coronal suture

Frontal bone

Corona radiata

Scalp

Diploe

Inner plate of parietal bone

Outer plate of parietal bone

Parietal lobe

Meningeal layer of dura mater

Dura mater

Superior sagittal sinus

Frontal lobe

Longitudinal fissure

Cerebral v.

Arachnoid mater

Subdural space

Falx cerebri

Parietal bone

Superior sagittal sinus

Transverse Section

The plane of section passes approximately 9 cm above the orbitomeatal line and includes the falx cerebri.

HEAD AND NECK
Plate 1 – 6

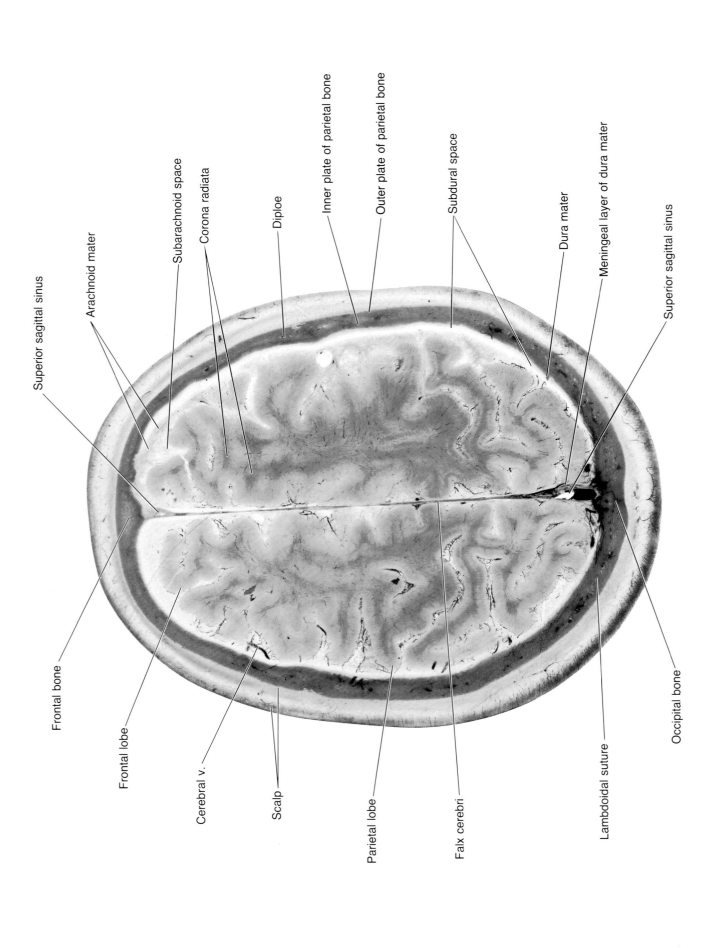

Superior sagittal sinus

Arachnoid mater

Subarachnoid space

Corona radiata

Diploe

Inner plate of parietal bone

Outer plate of parietal bone

Subdural space

Dura mater

Meningeal layer of dura mater

Superior sagittal sinus

Frontal bone

Frontal lobe

Cerebral v.

Scalp

Parietal lobe

Falx cerebri

Lambdoidal suture

Occipital bone

Transverse Section

The plane of section passes approximately 7.5 cm above the orbitomeatal line and includes the falx cerebri.

HEAD AND NECK
Plate 1 – 7

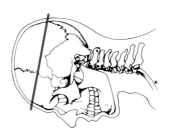

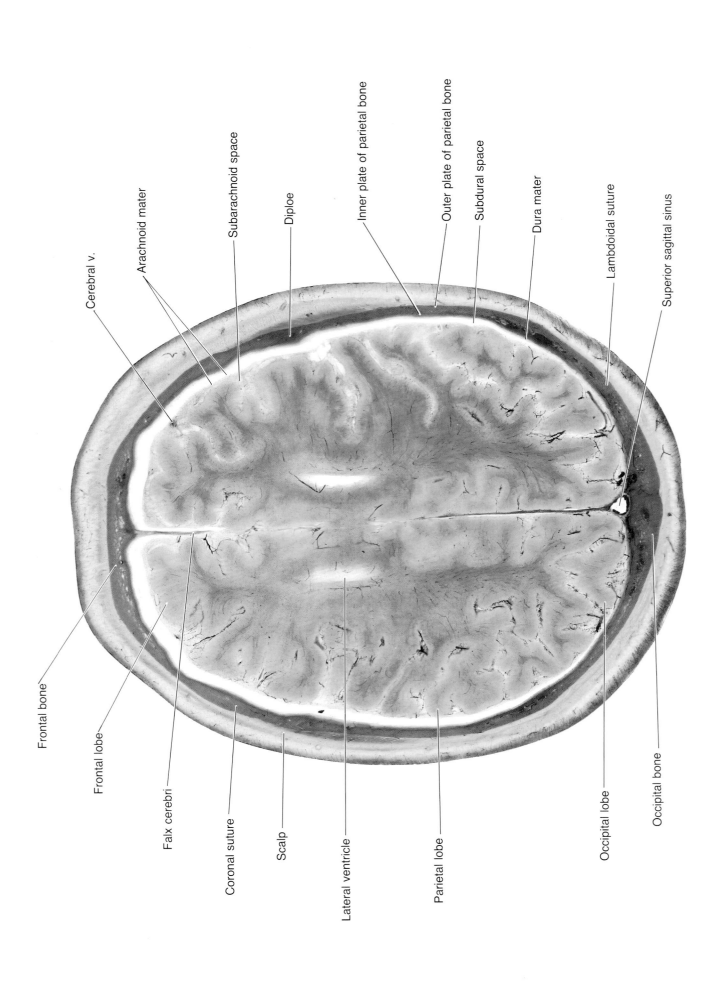

Cerebral v.

Arachnoid mater

Subarachnoid space

Diploe

Inner plate of parietal bone

Outer plate of parietal bone

Subdural space

Dura mater

Lambdoidal suture

Superior sagittal sinus

Frontal bone

Frontal lobe

Falx cerebri

Coronal suture

Scalp

Lateral ventricle

Parietal lobe

Occipital lobe

Occipital bone

The plane of section passes approximately 6.5 cm above the orbitomeatal line and includes a portion of the lateral ventricles.

Transverse Section

HEAD AND NECK
Plate 1 – 8

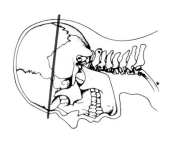

Glabella

Crista galli

Genu of corpus callosum

Middle meningeal a.

Septum pellucidum

Internal capsule

Fornix

Posterior horn of lateral ventricle

Falx cerebri

Diploe

Superior sagittal sinus

Frontal sinus

Frontal bone

Frontal lobe

Anterior horn of lateral ventricle

Head of caudate nucleus

Putamen

Temporalis m.

Superficial temporal vessels

Thalamus

Choroid plexus

Splenium of corpus callosum

Occipital lobe

Occipital bone

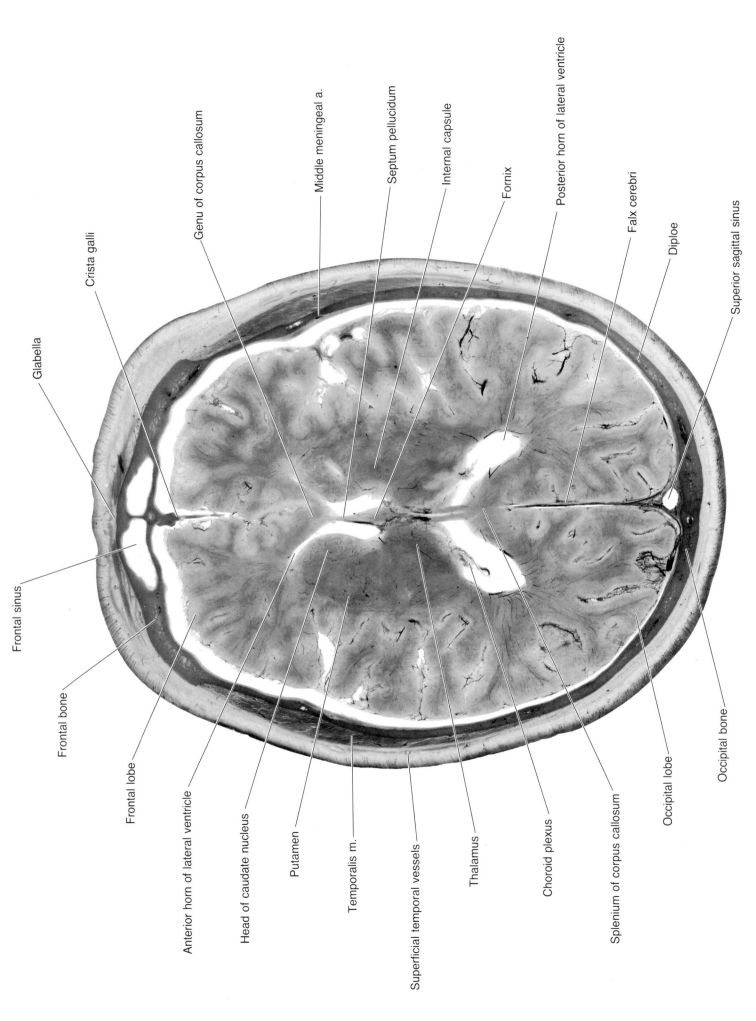

HEAD AND NECK
Plate 1 – 9

The plane of section passes approximately 6 cm above the orbitomeatal line and includes portions of the anterior and posterior horns of the lateral ventricles.

Transverse Section

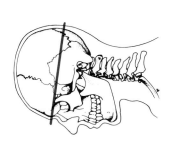

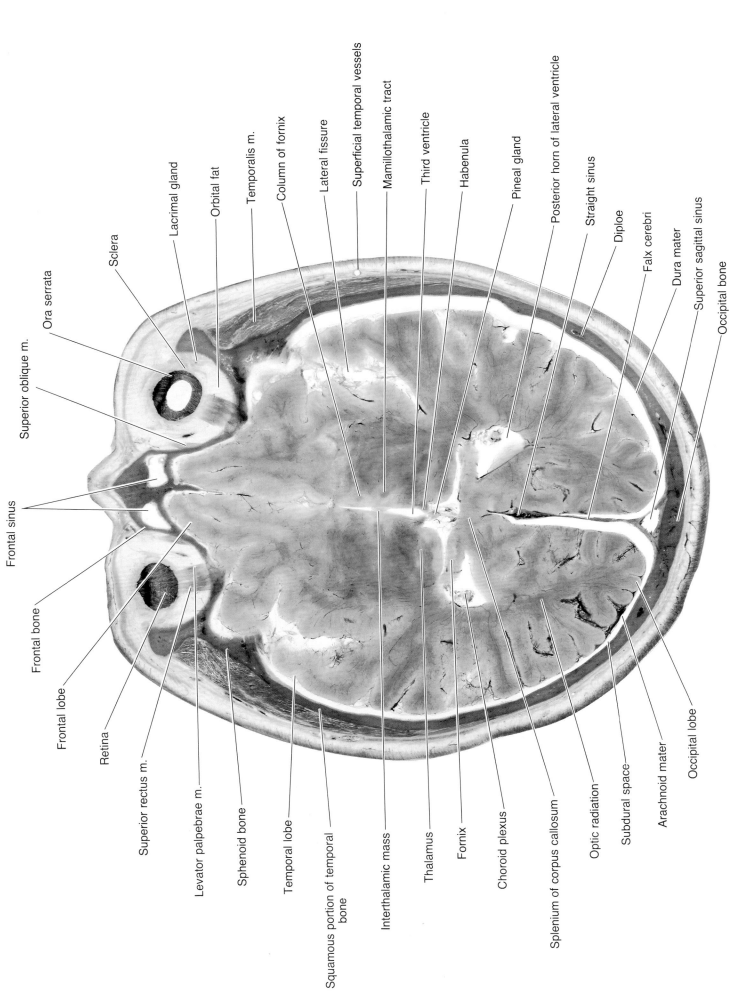

Frontal sinus

Superior oblique m.

Ora serrata

Sclera

Lacrimal gland

Orbital fat

Temporalis m.

Column of fornix

Lateral fissure

Superficial temporal vessels

Mamillothalamic tract

Third ventricle

Habenula

Pineal gland

Posterior horn of lateral ventricle

Straight sinus

Diploe

Falx cerebri

Dura mater

Superior sagittal sinus

Occipital bone

Frontal bone

Frontal lobe

Retina

Superior rectus m.

Levator palpebrae m.

Sphenoid bone

Temporal lobe

Squamous portion of temporal bone

Interthalamic mass

Thalamus

Fornix

Choroid plexus

Splenium of corpus callosum

Optic radiation

Subdural space

Arachnoid mater

Occipital lobe

HEAD AND NECK
Plate 1 – 10

The plane of section passes through the orbit approximately 3 cm above the orbitomeatal line and includes the superior aspect of the eyeball and a portion of the posterior horn of the lateral ventricle.

Transverse Section

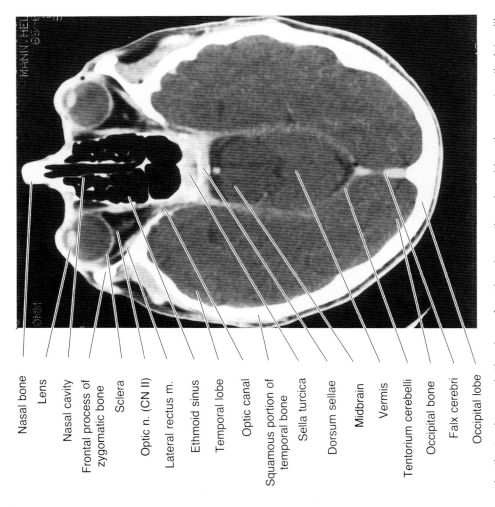

Nasal bone

Lens

Nasal cavity

Frontal process of
zygomatic bone

Sclera

Optic n. (CN II)

Lateral rectus m.

Ethmoid sinus

Temporal lobe

Optic canal

Squamous portion of
temporal bone

Sella turcica

Dorsum sellae

Midbrain

Vermis

Tentorium cerebelli

Occipital bone

Falx cerebri

Occipital lobe

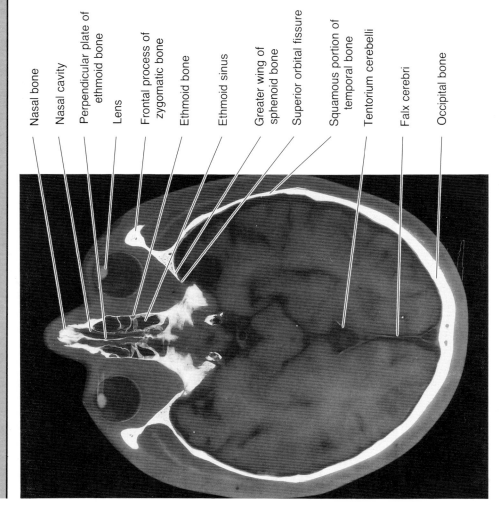

Nasal bone

Nasal cavity

Perpendicular plate of
ethmoid bone

Lens

Frontal process of
zygomatic bone

Ethmoid bone

Ethmoid sinus

Greater wing of
sphenoid bone

Superior orbital fissure

Squamous portion of
temporal bone

Tentorium cerebelli

Falx cerebri

Occipital bone

The sections shown in Plate 1-11 and the accompanying radiograph (Plate 1-11 Radiograph) and CT (Plate 1-11 CT) pass transversely through the skull and associated structures at the level of the orbit. The radiograph of the actual specimen shown in Plate 1-11 allows one to identify the bones of the skull at this level, especially those associated with the nasal cavity and orbit. Two of the most complex bones — the ethmoid and sphenoid — of the skull are present at this level. The ethmoid borders the anterior portion of the cranial cavity, the orbit, and the nasal cavity, and articulates with thirteen other bones (frontal, sphenoid, two nasals, two maxillae, two lacrimals, two palatines, two inferior nasal conchae, and the vomer). The thin walled cellular cavities which divide the ethmoid sinus into three groups of air cells — anterior, middle, and posterior — can be seen. At this plane of section, the perpendicular plate of the ethmoid forms the bony component of the nasal septum. Anteriorly, the ethmoid articulates with the nasal bones. Posteriorly, it articulates with the sphenoid bone.

The sphenoid is centrally positioned. It borders the cranial cavity, orbit, nasal cavity, and the upper posterior portion of the oral cavity and articulates with twelve bones (four unpaired — the vomer, ethmoid, frontal, and occipital; and four paired — the temporal, parietal, zygomatic, and palatine). The superior orbital fissure, the opening between the greater and lesser wings of the sphenoid bone, can readily be seen on the left side by comparing the radiograph with the specimen. The opening of the optic canal within the lesser wing of the sphenoid can also be visualized by

comparing the two images. In the plane of section shown, the sphenoid can be seen to articulate with the zygomatic bone, laterally, and with the squamous portion of the temporal bone, posteriorly. The occipital bone can be seen in the posterior portion of the section.

The plane of section passes through the eyes at the level of the lens. The optic nerve can be seen as it passes from the optic chiasma, through the optic canal, and to the eye. Within the orbit the optic nerve is surrounded by periorbital fat. Two of the ocular muscles can be identified — the Lateral rectus and the Medial rectus. A branch of the oculomotor nerve can be seen as it passes through the orbit to reach the medial rectus muscle. A number of structures, including the lacrimal glands and sacs, branches of the ophthalmic artery, conjunctival sac, and Orbicularis oculi muscle, can be identified in the orbit and in association with the eye.

The section passes through the brain and arteries associated with the circle of Willis, namely the internal carotid, middle cerebral, and basilar arteries. In this same region, the infundibulum can be seen immediately posterior to the optic chiasma. The CT represents a different plane and shows much more of the cerebellum.

Plate 1-11 Radiograph
Transverse Section

Plate 1-11 CT
Transverse Section

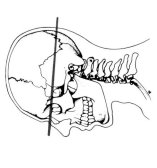

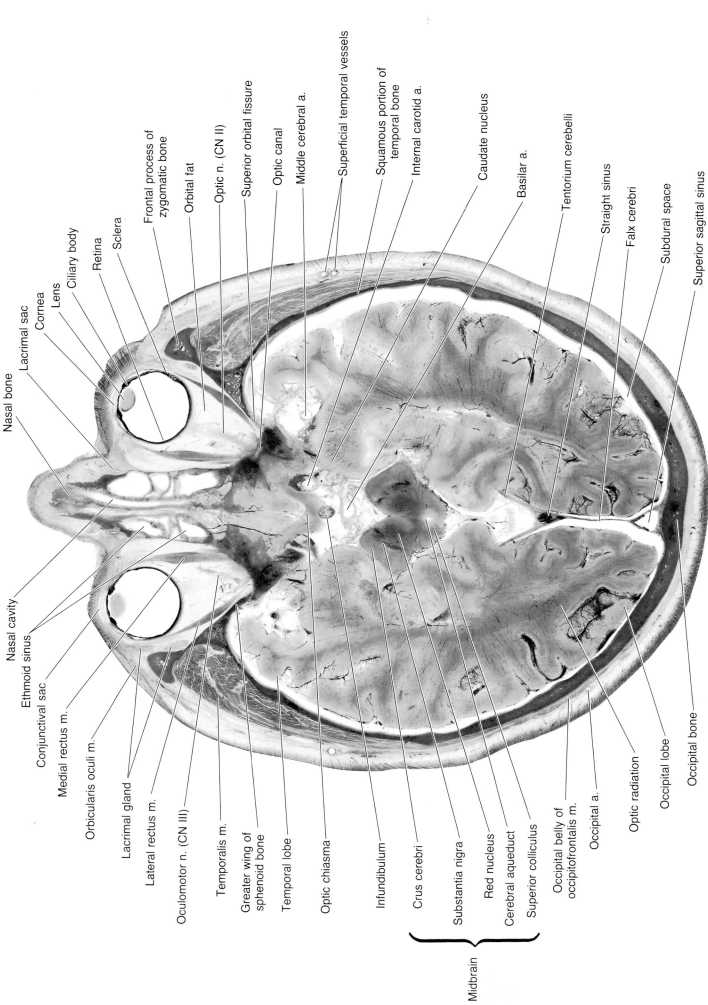

Nasal bone

Lacrimal sac

Cornea

Lens

Ciliary body

Retina

Sclera

Frontal process of zygomatic bone

Orbital fat

Optic n. (CN II)

Superior orbital fissure

Optic canal

Middle cerebral a.

Superficial temporal vessels

Squamous portion of temporal bone

Internal carotid a.

Caudate nucleus

Basilar a.

Tentorium cerebelli

Straight sinus

Falx cerebri

Subdural space

Superior sagittal sinus

Ethmoid sinus

Conjunctival sac

Medial rectus m.

Orbicularis oculi m.

Nasal cavity

Lacrimal gland

Lateral rectus m.

Oculomotor n. (CN III)

Temporalis m.

Greater wing of sphenoid bone

Temporal lobe

Optic chiasma

Infundibulum

Crus cerebri

Substantia nigra

Red nucleus

Cerebral aqueduct

Superior colliculus

Occipital belly of occipitofrontalis m.

Occipital a.

Optic radiation

Occipital lobe

Occipital bone

Midbrain

HEAD AND NECK
Plate 1 – 11

The plane of section passes through the orbit approximately 1.5 cm above the orbitomeatal line and includes the lens of the eye, optic chiasma and infundibulum.

Transverse Section

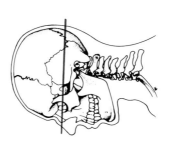

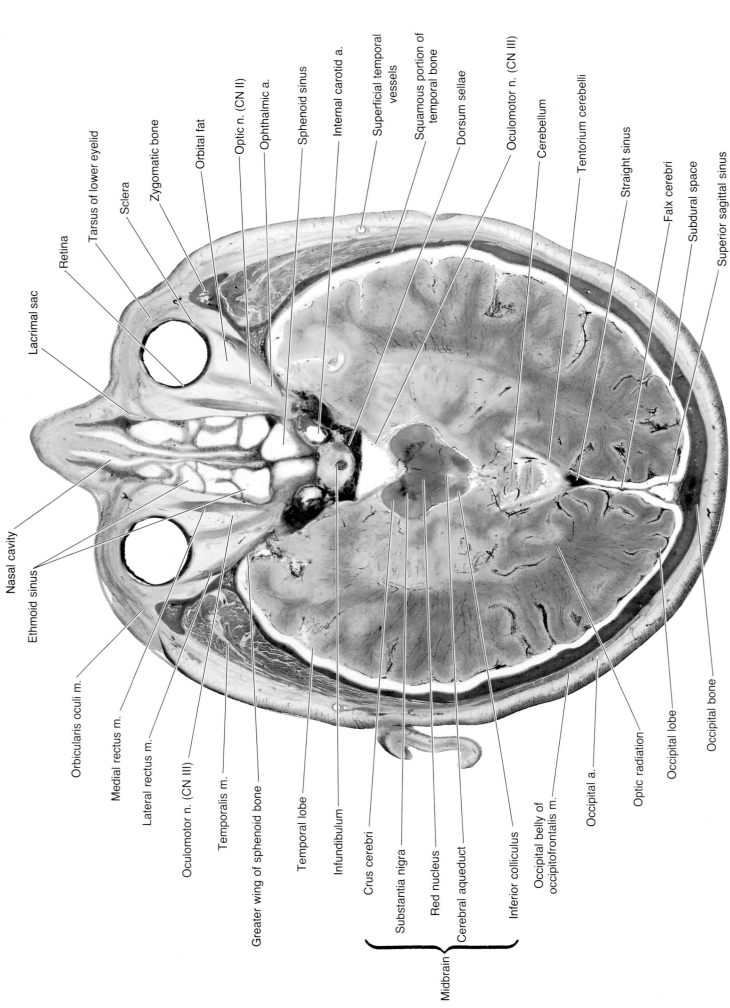

Nasal cavity

Ethmoid sinus

Lacrimal sac

Retina

Tarsus of lower eyelid

Sclera

Zygomatic bone

Orbital fat

Optic n. (CN II)

Ophthalmic a.

Sphenoid sinus

Internal carotid a.

Superficial temporal vessels

Squamous portion of temporal bone

Dorsum sellae

Oculomotor n. (CN III)

Cerebellum

Tentorium cerebelli

Straight sinus

Falx cerebri

Subdural space

Superior sagittal sinus

Orbicularis oculi m.

Medial rectus m.

Lateral rectus m.

Oculomotor n. (CN III)

Temporalis m.

Greater wing of sphenoid bone

Temporal lobe

Infundibulum

Crus cerebri

Substantia nigra

Red nucleus

Cerebral aqueduct

Inferior colliculus

Midbrain

Occipital belly of occipitofrontalis m.

Occipital a.

Optic radiation

Occipital lobe

Occipital bone

HEAD AND NECK
Plate 1 – 12

The plane of section passes through the orbit approximately 1 cm above the orbitomeatal line and includes the optic nerve. Portions of the sphenoid and ethmoid sinuses are included in the section.

Transverse Section

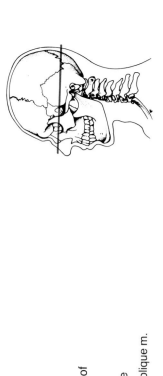

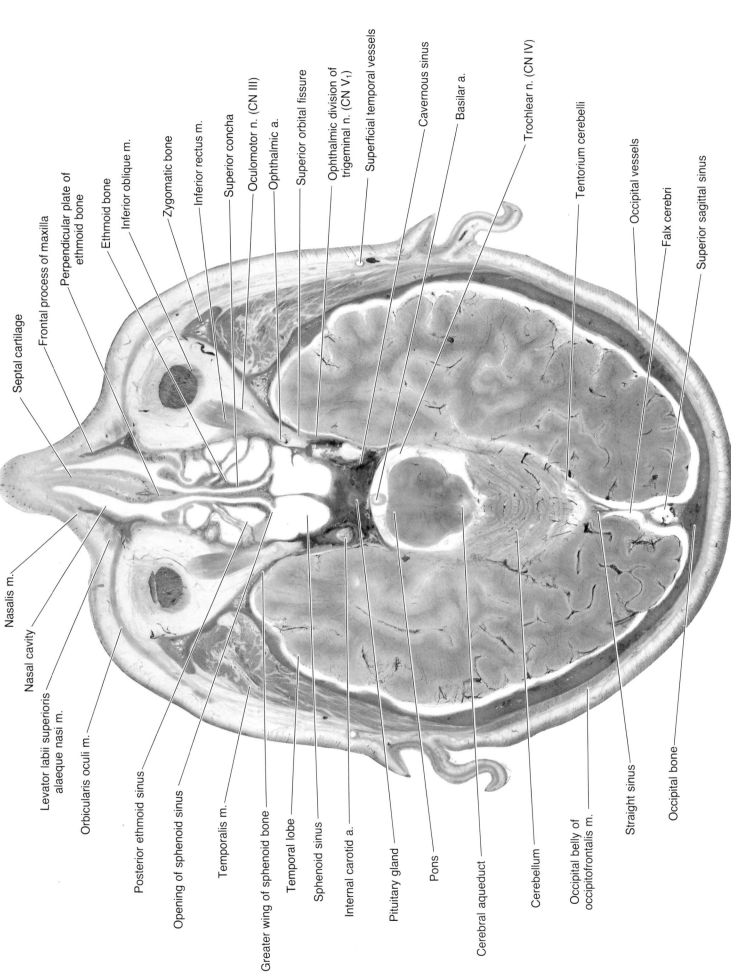

Septal cartilage

Frontal process of maxilla

Perpendicular plate of ethmoid bone

Ethmoid bone

Inferior oblique m.

Zygomatic bone

Inferior rectus m.

Superior concha

Oculomotor n. (CN III)

Ophthalmic a.

Superior orbital fissure

Ophthalmic division of trigeminal n. (CN V₁)

Superficial temporal vessels

Cavernous sinus

Basilar a.

Trochlear n. (CN IV)

Tentorium cerebelli

Occipital vessels

Falx cerebri

Superior sagittal sinus

Nasalis m.

Nasal cavity

Levator labii superioris alaeque nasi m.

Orbicularis oculi m.

Posterior ethmoid sinus

Opening of sphenoid sinus

Temporalis m.

Greater wing of sphenoid bone

Temporal lobe

Sphenoid sinus

Internal carotid a.

Pituitary gland

Pons

Cerebral aqueduct

Cerebellum

Occipital belly of occipitofrontalis m.

Straight sinus

Occipital bone

Transverse Section

The plane of section passes through the orbit approximately 0.5 cm above the orbitomeatal line. Pituitary gland and portions of sphenoid and ethmoid sinuses are included in the section.

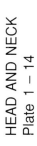

Nasalis m.

Levator labii superioris
alaeque nasi m.

Superior concha

Orbicularis oculi m.

Inferior oblique m.

Inferior rectus m.

Oculomotor n. (CN III)

Maxillary bone

Maxillary sinus

Sphenoid sinus

Temporalis m.

Squamous portion of
temporal bone

Basilar portion of
occipital bone

Cavernous sinus

Pons

Superior cerebellar
peduncle

Cerebellum

Straight sinus

Occipital vessels

Occipital bone

Nasal cavity

Frontal process of maxilla

Septal cartilage

Nasolacrimal duct

Perpendicular plate of
ethmoid bone

Ethmoid bulla

Middle ethmoid air cell

Zygomatic process of
zygomatic bone

Middle concha

Infraorbital n.

Vomer

Superficial temporal
vessels

Internal carotid a.

Trigeminal n. (CN V)

Basilar a.

Fourth ventricle

Lambdoid suture

Superior sagittal sinus

HEAD AND NECK
Plate 1 – 14

The plane of section passes through the floor of the orbit and includes the inferior oblique and rectus muscles.
Portions of the sphenoid and ethmoid sinuses are included in the section.

Transverse Section

Nasal cavity

Septal cartilage

Levator labii superioris
alaeque nasi m.

Lacrimal bone

Nasolacrimal duct

Infraorbital n.

Middle concha

Pterygomaxillary fissure

Maxillary division of
trigeminal n. (CN V₂)

Foramen rotundum

Sphenoid sinus

Internal carotid a.

Trigeminal ganglion

Superficial temporal vessels

Basilar portion
of occipital bone

Basilar a.

Cochlea

Anterior semicircular canal

Trigeminal n. (CN V)

Superior cerebellar peduncle

Fourth ventricle

Cerebellum

Confluence of superior
sagittal and straight sinuses

Internal occipital protuberance

Nasalis m.

Maxillary bone

Maxillary sinus

Zygomatic bone

Sphenopalatine foramen

Zygomatic process of
temporal bone

Maxillary a.

Pterygopalatine fossa

Sphenopalatine a.

Temporal lobe

Squamous portion of
temporal bone

Mastoid air cells

Petrous portion of
temporal bone

Anterior semicircular canal

Middle cerebellar peduncle

Pons

Transverse sinus

Tentorium cerebelli

Occipital lobe

Occipital bone

HEAD AND NECK
Plate 1 – 15

The plane of section passes through the petrous portion of the temporal bone and includes portions of the cochlea and
anterior semicircular canal. Pterygopalatine fossa is included in the section.

Transverse Section

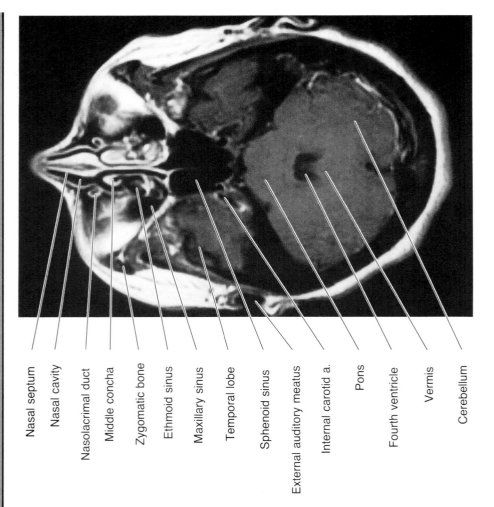

Nasal septum
Nasal cavity
Nasolacrimal duct
Middle concha
Zygomatic bone
Ethmoid sinus
Maxillary sinus
Temporal lobe
Sphenoid sinus
External auditory meatus
Internal carotid a.
Pons
Fourth ventricle
Vermis
Cerebellum

Section 1-16 passes through the zygomatic arch and includes part of the superior aspect of the infratemporal fossa. The pterygomaxillary fissure can be identified as it leads medially into the pterygopalatine fossa. The vertical plate of the palatine bone can be identified as it forms the medial wall of the pterygopalatine fossa and contributes to the lateral wall of the nasal cavity. Portions of the third part of the maxillary artery can be seen in the pterygopalatine fossa.

Posteriorly, the sections shown in Plates 1-16 and 1-16 CT pass obliquely through the tentorium cerebelli, such that portions of the occipital lobes, cerebellum, pons, and fourth ventricle are included in the section. In Plate 1-16 the section includes the right transverse dural sinus. In all three Plates, the basal artery can be seen as it lies anterior to the pons and posterior to the basilar portion of the occipital bone.

Plate 1-16 MRI
Transverse Section

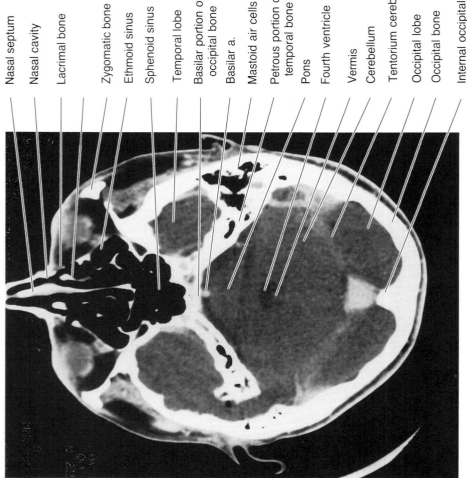

Nasal septum
Nasal cavity
Lacrimal bone
Zygomatic bone
Ethmoid sinus
Sphenoid sinus
Temporal lobe
Basilar portion of occipital bone
Basilar a.
Mastoid air cells
Petrous portion of temporal bone
Pons
Fourth ventricle
Vermis
Cerebellum
Tentorium cerebelli
Occipital lobe
Occipital bone
Internal occipital protuberance

The sections shown in Plate 1-16 and the accompanying CT (Plate 1-16 CT) and MRI (Plate 1-16 MRI) pass through the petrous portion of the temporal bone and include portions of the cochlea and semicircular canals of the inner ear. In Plate 1-16 the internal auditory meatus is included in the section. The CT and MRI plates are at a slightly different plane and do include the internal auditory meatus. In all three plates the inferior portion of the left and right temporal lobes are included in the section as they lie in the floor of the middle cranial fossa. Medial to the temporal lobes the sphenoid sinus and adjacent internal carotid arteries can be seen.

In the nasal cavity the sections pass through the middle concha. The nasolacrimal duct lies in the anterolateral wall of the nasal cavity. In Plates 1-16 and 1-16 MRI the nasolacrimal duct is clearly visible within the lacrimal bone as it borders the maxillary sinus and nasal cavity at the level shown. Superior to the level shown, the lacrimal bone borders the orbit and nasal cavity (see Plate 1-14).

Plate 1-16 CT
Transverse Section

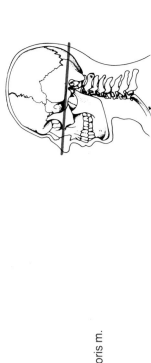

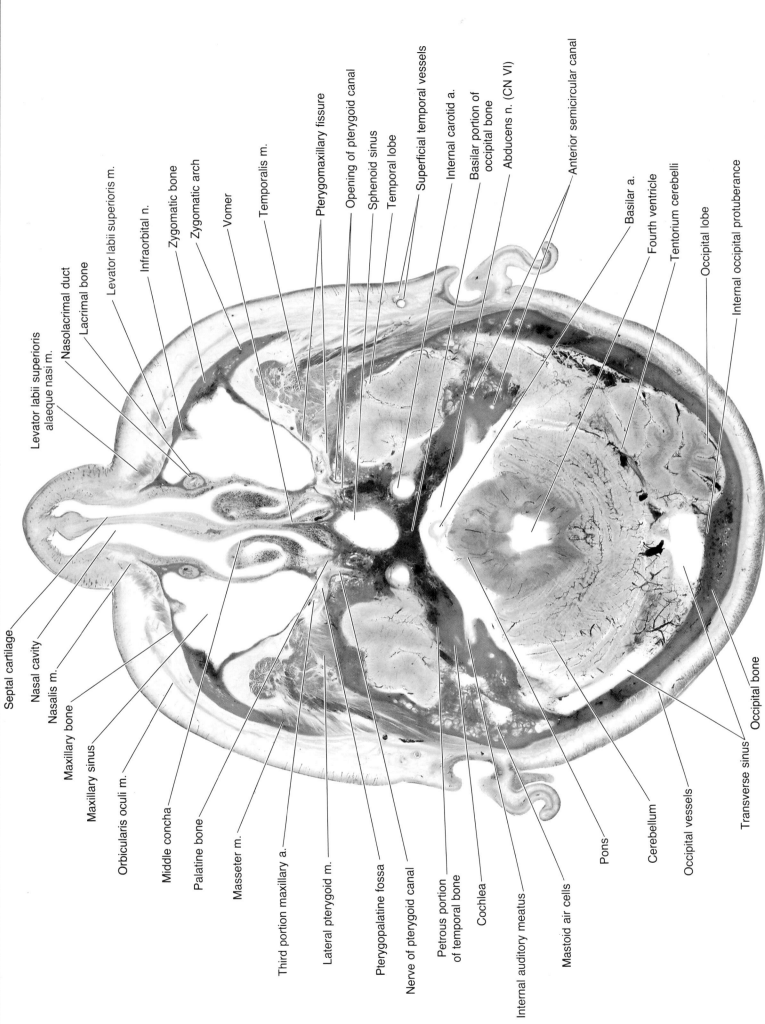

Septal cartilage

Nasal cavity

Nasalis m.

Maxillary bone

Levator labii superioris
alaeque nasi m.

Nasolacrimal duct

Lacrimal bone

Levator labii superioris m.

Infraorbital n.

Zygomatic bone

Zygomatic arch

Vomer

Temporalis m.

Pterygomaxillary fissure

Opening of pterygoid canal

Sphenoid sinus

Temporal lobe

Superficial temporal vessels

Internal carotid a.

Basilar portion of
occipital bone

Abducens n. (CN VI)

Anterior semicircular canal

Basilar a.

Fourth ventricle

Tentorium cerebelli

Occipital lobe

Internal occipital protuberance

Maxillary sinus

Orbicularis oculi m.

Middle concha

Palatine bone

Masseter m.

Third portion maxillary a.

Lateral pterygoid m.

Pterygopalatine fossa

Nerve of pterygoid canal

Petrous portion
of temporal bone

Cochlea

Internal auditory meatus

Mastoid air cells

Pons

Cerebellum

Occipital vessels

Transverse sinus

Occipital bone

Transverse Section

The plane of section passes through the petrous portion of the temporal bone and includes portions of the cochlea
and anterior semicircular canal. Internal auditory meatus is included in the section.

HEAD AND NECK
Plate 1 – 16

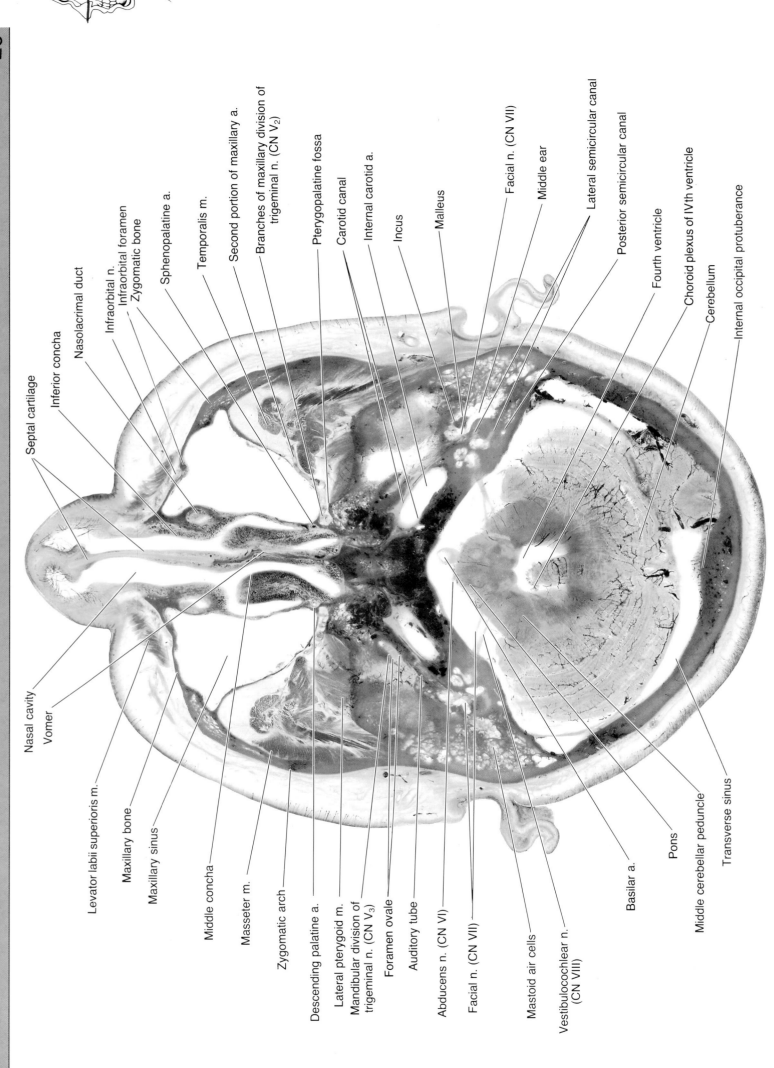

Nasal cavity

Vomer

Septal cartilage

Inferior concha

Nasolacrimal duct

Levator labii superioris m.

Maxillary bone

Maxillary sinus

Infraorbital n.
Infraorbital foramen
Zygomatic bone

Sphenopalatine a.

Temporalis m.

Second portion of maxillary a.

Branches of maxillary division of
trigeminal n. (CN V₂)

Pterygopalatine fossa

Carotid canal

Internal carotid a.

Incus

Malleus

Facial n. (CN VII)

Middle ear

Lateral semicircular canal

Posterior semicircular canal

Fourth ventricle

Choroid plexus of IVth ventricle

Cerebellum

Internal occipital protuberance

Middle concha

Masseter m.

Zygomatic arch

Descending palatine a.

Lateral pterygoid m.

Mandibular division of
trigeminal n. (CN V₃)

Foramen ovale

Auditory tube

Abducens n. (CN VI)

Facial n. (CN VII)

Mastoid air cells

Vestibulocochlear n.
(CN VIII)

Basilar a.

Pons

Middle cerebellar peduncle

Transverse sinus

The plane of section passes through the petrous portion of the temporal bone and includes the carotid canal
and portions of the lateral and posterior semicircular canals.

Transverse Section

HEAD AND NECK
Plate 1 – 17

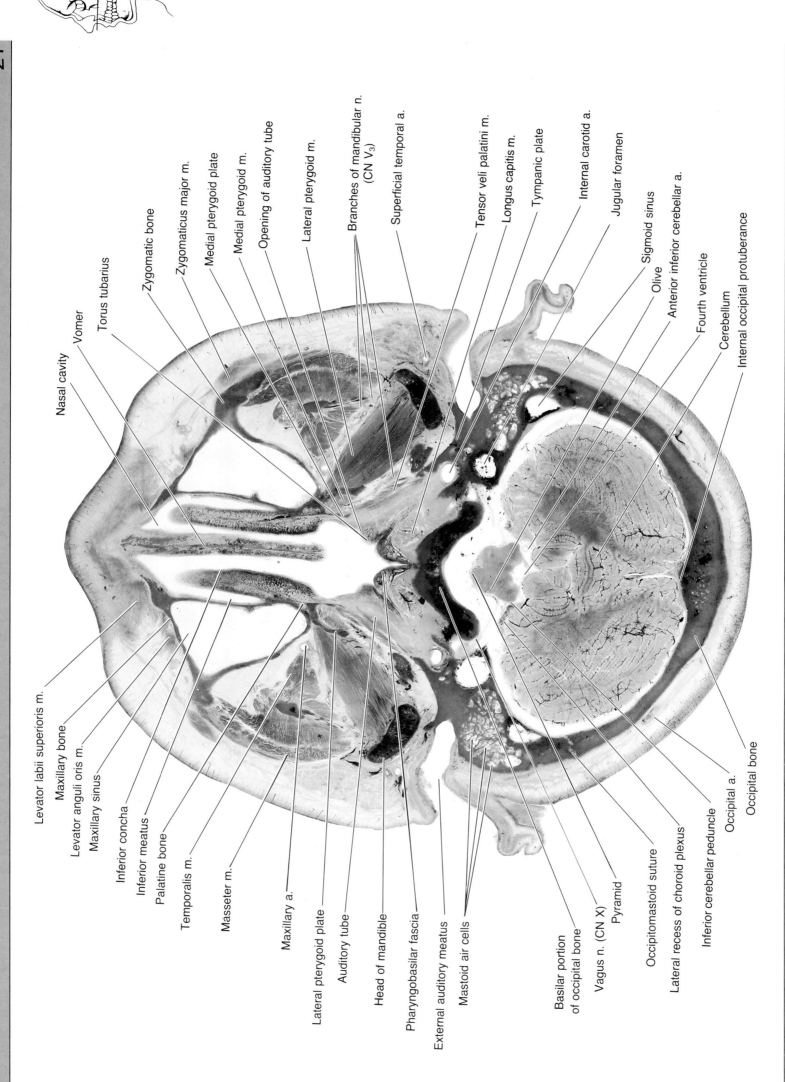

Levator labii superioris m.

Maxillary bone

Levator anguli oris m.

Maxillary sinus

Inferior concha

Inferior meatus

Palatine bone

Temporalis m.

Masseter m.

Maxillary a.

Lateral pterygoid plate

Auditory tube

Head of mandible

Pharyngobasilar fascia

External auditory meatus

Mastoid air cells

Basilar portion
of occipital bone

Vagus n. (CN X)

Pyramid

Occipitomastoid suture

Lateral recess of choroid plexus

Inferior cerebellar peduncle

Occipital a.

Occipital bone

Nasal cavity

Vomer

Torus tubarius

Zygomatic bone

Zygomaticus major m.

Medial pterygoid plate

Medial pterygoid m.

Opening of auditory tube

Lateral pterygoid m.

Branches of mandibular n.
(CN V₃)

Superficial temporal a.

Tensor veli palatini m.

Longus capitis m.

Tympanic plate

Internal carotid a.

Jugular foramen

Sigmoid sinus

Olive

Anterior inferior cerebellar a.

Fourth ventricle

Cerebellum

Internal occipital protuberance

Transverse Section

The plane of section passes through the petrous portion of the temporal bone and includes mastoid air cells. The head
of the mandible and branches of the mandibular nerve are included in the section.

HEAD AND NECK
Plate 1 – 18

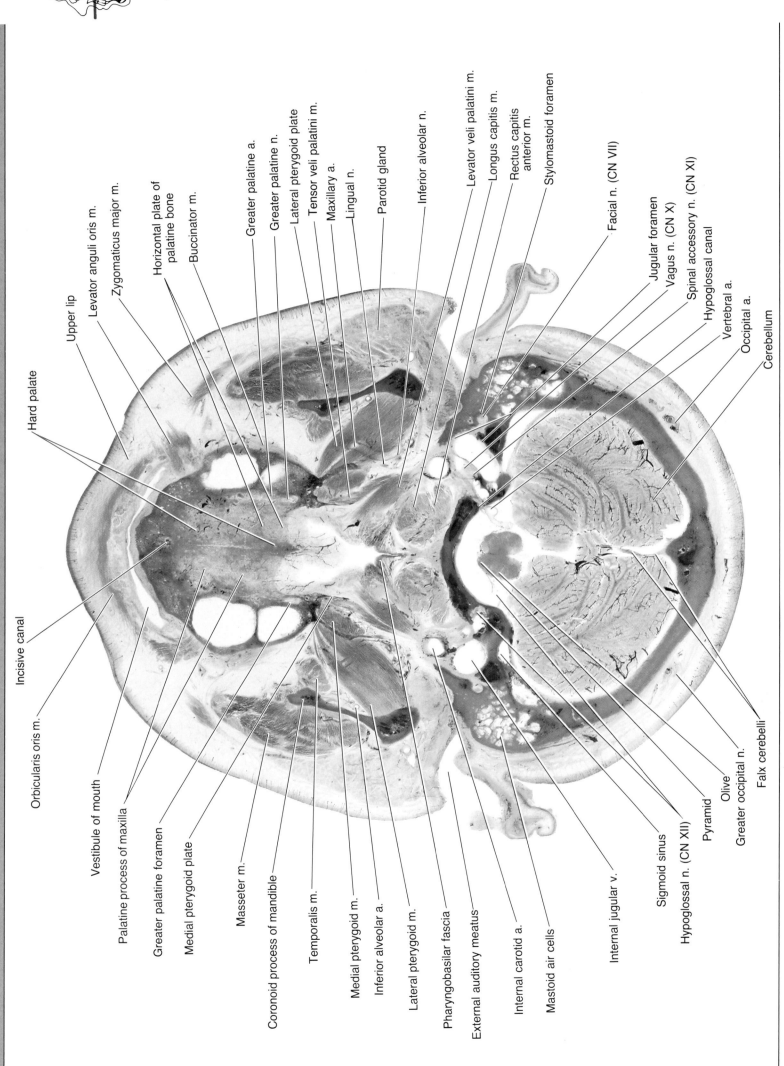

Incisive canal

Hard palate

Upper lip

Levator anguli oris m.

Zygomaticus major m.

Horizontal plate of palatine bone

Buccinator m.

Greater palatine a.

Greater palatine n.

Lateral pterygoid plate

Tensor veli palatini m.

Maxillary a.

Lingual n.

Parotid gland

Inferior alveolar n.

Levator veli palatini m.

Longus capitis m.

Rectus capitis anterior m.

Stylomastoid foramen

Facial n. (CN VII)

Jugular foramen

Vagus n. (CN X)

Spinal accessory n. (CN XI)

Hypoglossal canal

Vertebral a.

Occipital a.

Cerebellum

Orbicularis oris m.

Vestibule of mouth

Palatine process of maxilla

Greater palatine foramen

Medial pterygoid plate

Masseter m.

Coronoid process of mandible

Temporalis m.

Medial pterygoid m.

Inferior alveolar a.

Lateral pterygoid m.

Pharyngobasilar fascia

External auditory meatus

Internal carotid a.

Mastoid air cells

Internal jugular v.

Sigmoid sinus

Hypoglossal n. (CN XII)

Pyramid

Olive

Greater occipital n.

Falx cerebelli

The plane of section passes through the hard palate and the mastoid process.
The jugular foramen and the hypoglossal canal are included in the section.

Transverse Section

HEAD AND NECK
Plate 1 – 19

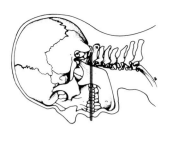

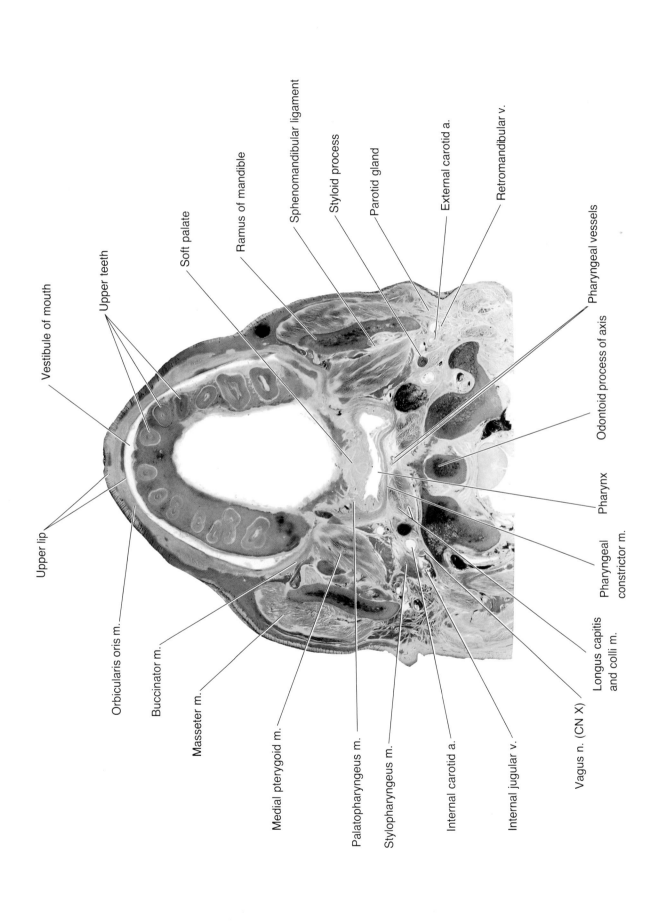

Vestibule of mouth

Upper teeth

Soft palate

Ramus of mandible

Sphenomandibular ligament

Styloid process

Parotid gland

External carotid a.

Retromandibular v.

Pharyngeal vessels

Upper lip

Orbicularis oris m.

Buccinator m.

Masseter m.

Medial pterygoid m.

Palatopharyngeus m.

Stylopharyngeus m.

Internal carotid a.

Internal jugular v.

Vagus n. (CN X)

Longus capitis and colli m.

Pharyngeal constrictor m.

Pharynx

Odontoid process of axis

HEAD AND NECK
Plate 1 – 20

The plane of section passes through the upper teeth, ramus of the mandible, and odontoid process of the axis.
Portions of the oral cavity, vestibule of the mouth, and pharynx are included in the section.

Transverse Section

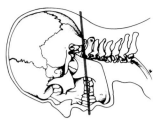

Upper lip

Levator anguli oris m.

Masseter m.

Inferior alveolar n.

Parotid duct

Ramus of mandible

External carotid a.

Parotid gland

Internal carotid a.

Styloid process

Rectus capitis anterior m.

Mastoid process

Posterior belly of digastric m.

Posterior auricular a.

Portion of atlas

Condyle

Vertebral a.

Occipital a.

Odontoid process of axis

Greater occipital n.

Oropharynx

Zygomaticus major m.

Buccinator m.

Medial pterygoid m.

Lingual n.

Inferior alveolar n.

Inferior alveolar a.

Pharyngeal constrictor m.

Pharyngeal vessels

Longus capitis and colli m.

Vagal ganglion

Hypoglossal n. (CN XII)

Facial n. (CN VII)

Internal jugular v.

Sternocleidomastoid m.

Rectus capitis lateralis m.

Longissimus capitis m.

Pyramid of medulla oblongata

Splenius capitis m.

Obliquus capitis superior m.

Semispinalis capitis m.

Cerebellum

Occipital bone

The plane of section passes through the tongue, ramus of the mandible, mastoid process, styloid process, and condyles.
Portions of the oral cavity and oropharynx are included in the section.

Transverse Section

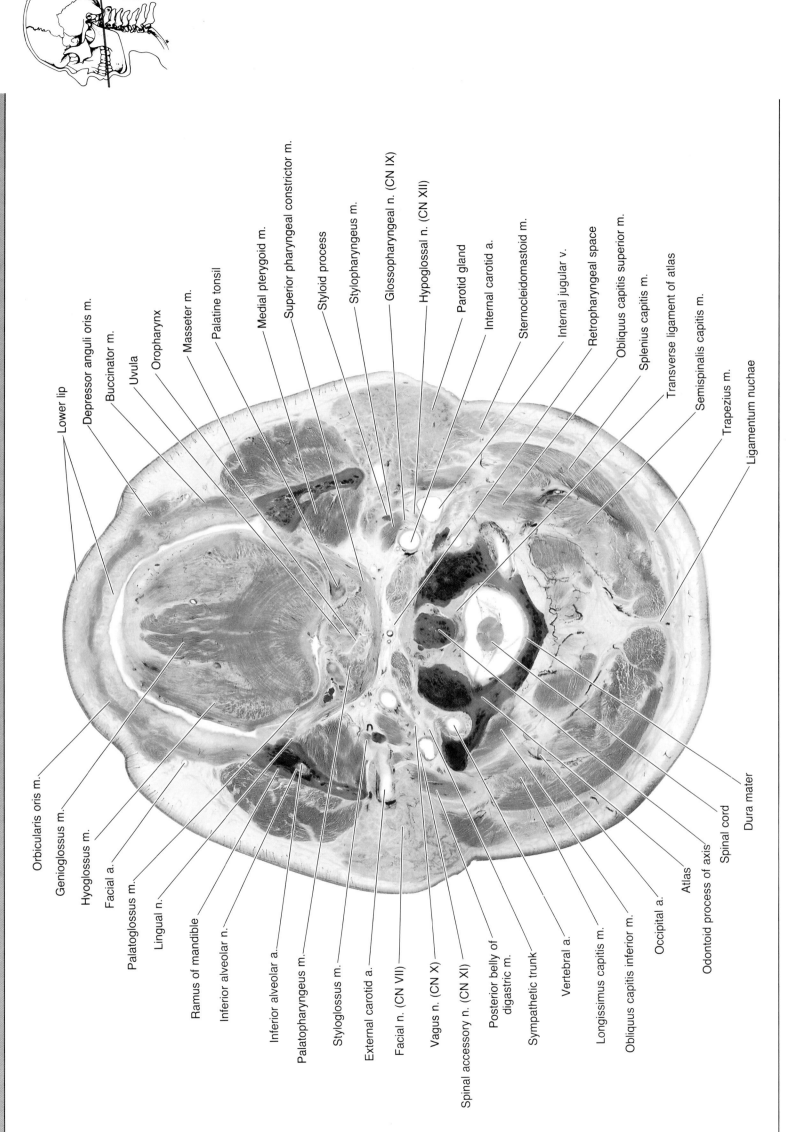

- Orbicularis oris m.
- Genioglossus m.
- Hyoglossus m.
- Facial a.
- Palatoglossus m.
- Lingual n.
- Ramus of mandible
- Inferior alveolar n.
- Inferior alveolar a.
- Palatopharyngeus m.
- Styloglossus m.
- External carotid a.
- Facial n. (CN VII)
- Vagus n. (CN X)
- Spinal accessory n. (CN XI)
- Posterior belly of digastric m.
- Sympathetic trunk
- Vertebral a.
- Longissimus capitis m.
- Obliquus capitis inferior m.
- Occipital a.
- Odontoid process of axis
- Atlas
- Spinal cord
- Dura mater

- Lower lip
- Depressor anguli oris m.
- Buccinator m.
- Uvula
- Oropharynx
- Masseter m.
- Palatine tonsil
- Medial pterygoid m.
- Superior pharyngeal constrictor m.
- Styloid process
- Stylopharyngeus m.
- Glossopharyngeal n. (CN IX)
- Hypoglossal n. (CN XII)
- Parotid gland
- Internal carotid a.
- Sternocleidomastoid m.
- Internal jugular v.
- Retropharyngeal space
- Obliquus capitis superior m.
- Splenius capitis m.
- Transverse ligament of atlas
- Semispinalis capitis m.
- Trapezius m.
- Ligamentum nuchae

The plane of section passes through the tongue, ramus of the mandible, styloid process, odontoid process of the axis, and portions of the atlas. The oropharynx is included in the section.

Transverse Section

HEAD AND NECK
Plate 1 – 22

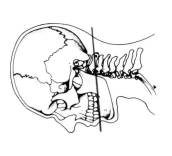

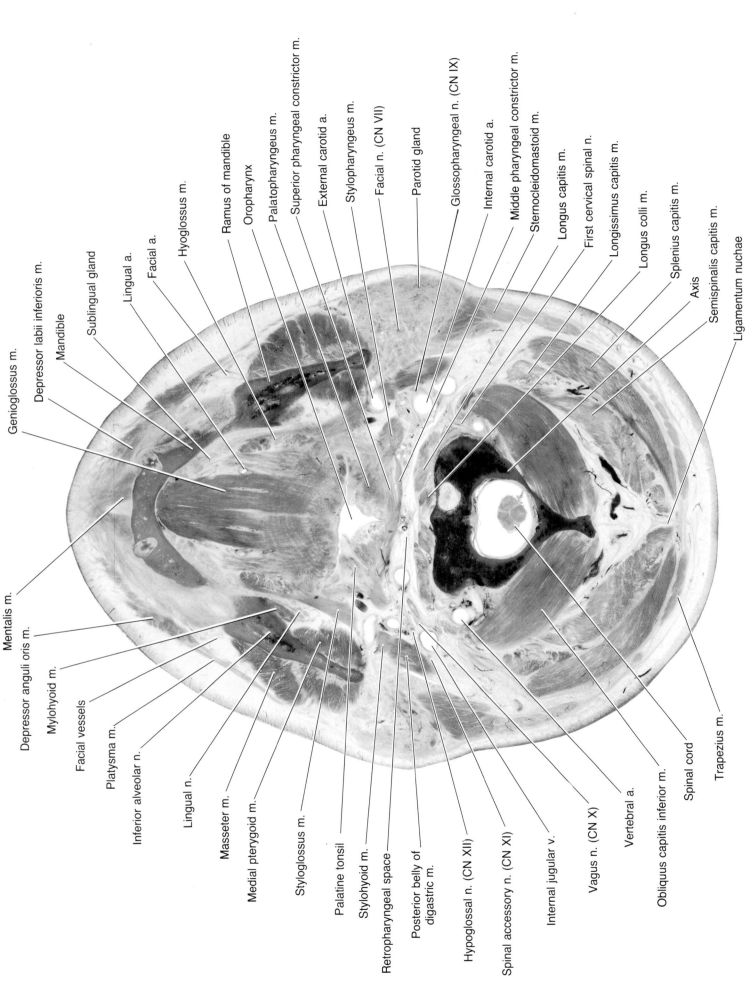

Mentalis m.

Genioglossus m.

Depressor labii inferioris m.

Depressor anguli oris m.

Mandible

Mylohyoid m.

Sublingual gland

Facial vessels

Lingual a.

Platysma m.

Facial a.

Inferior alveolar n.

Hyoglossus m.

Lingual n.

Ramus of mandible

Masseter m.

Oropharynx

Medial pterygoid m.

Palatopharyngeus m.

Styloglossus m.

Superior pharyngeal constrictor m.

Palatine tonsil

External carotid a.

Stylohyoid m.

Stylopharyngeus m.

Retropharyngeal space

Facial n. (CN VII)

Posterior belly of digastric m.

Parotid gland

Hypoglossal n. (CN XII)

Glossopharyngeal n. (CN IX)

Spinal accessory n. (CN XI)

Internal carotid a.

Internal jugular v.

Middle pharyngeal constrictor m.

Vagus n. (CN X)

Sternocleidomastoid m.

Vertebral a.

Longus capitis m.

Obliquus capitis inferior m.

First cervical spinal n.

Spinal cord

Longissimus capitis m.

Trapezius m.

Longus colli m.

Splenius capitis m.

Axis

Semispinalis capitis m.

Ligamentum nuchae

The plane of section passes through the mandible, floor of the oral cavity, and the axis. Portions of the styloglossus, hyoglossus, genioglossus, and mylohyoid muscles are included in the section.

Transverse Section

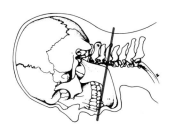

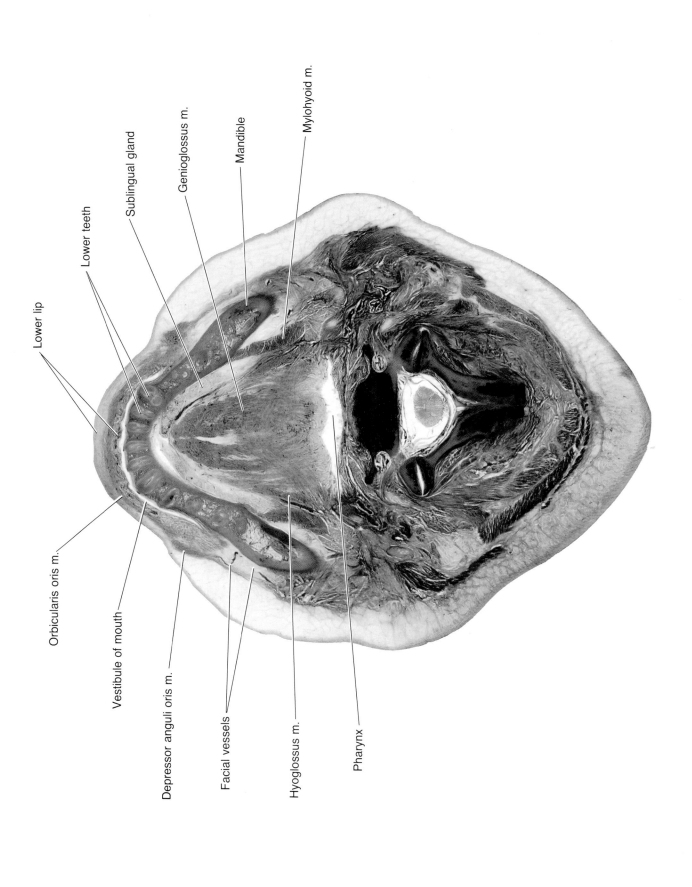

Lower lip

Lower teeth

Sublingual gland

Genioglossus m.

Mandible

Mylohyoid m.

Orbicularis oris m.

Vestibule of mouth

Depressor anguli oris m.

Facial vessels

Hyoglossus m.

Pharynx

The plane of section passes through the lower teeth, mandible, and floor of the oral cavity. Portions of the mylohyoid, hyoglossus, and genioglossus muscles are included in the section.

Transverse Section

Mentalis m.

Mandible

Mylohyoid m.

Hypoglossal n. (CN XII)

Lingual a.

Hyoglossus m.

Facial a.

Pharynx

Hypoglossal n. (CN XII)

Palatopharyngeus m.

Middle pharyngeal constrictor m.

Inferior pharyngeal constrictor m.

External carotid a.

Vagus n. (CN X)

Internal jugular v.

Spinal accessory n. (CN XI)

Vertebral a.

Spinal n.

Levator scapulae m.

Longissimus capitis m.

Third cervical vertebra

Splenius capitis m.

Trapezius m.

Geniohyoid m.

Depressor labii inferioris m.

Genioglossus m.

Depressor anguli oris m.

Submandibular duct

Platysma m.

Facial vessels

Submandibular gland

Lingual tonsil

Stylohyoid m.

Posterior belly of digastric m.

Parotid gland

Sternocleidomastoid m.

Internal carotid a.

Longus capitis m.

Longus colli m.

Portion of axis

Intervertebral disc

Semispinalis cervicis m.

Semispinalis capitis m.

Ligamentum nuchae

Transverse Section

HEAD AND NECK
Plate 1 – 25

The plane of section passes through the lower border of the mandible and the third cervical vertebra. Portions of the axis, or second cervical vertebra, are included in the section.

Lymph node

Platysma m.

Mylohyoid m.

Central tendon of digastric m.

Submandibular gland

Thyroid cartilage

Pharyngeal raphe

Superior thyroid a.

Parotid gland

Common carotid a.

Internal jugular v.

Vagus n. (CN X)

Retropharyngeal space

Longus capitis m.

Longus colli m.

Scalenus medius m.

Levator scapulae m.

Vertebral a.

Spinal n.

Semispinalis cervicis m.

Semispinalis capitis m.

Splenius capitis m.

Ligamentum flavum

Intervertebral disc

Geniohyoid m.

Anterior belly of digastric m.

Body of hyoid bone

Lesser horn of hyoid bone

Epiglottic cartilage

Greater horn of hyoid bone

Laryngopharynx

Superior cornu of thyroid cartilage

Palatopharyngeus m.

Retromandibular v.

Sternocleidomastoid m.

Lymph nodes

Spinal accessory n. (CN XI)

Inferior pharyngeal constrictor m.

Longissimus cervicis m.

Body of third cervical vertebra

Longissimus capitis m.

Fourth cervical vertebra

Trapezius m.

Ligamentum nuchae

Transverse Section

The plane of section passes through the hyoid bone, superior cornu of the thyroid cartilage, and fourth cervical vertebra. Epiglottic cartilage and laryngopharynx are included in the section.

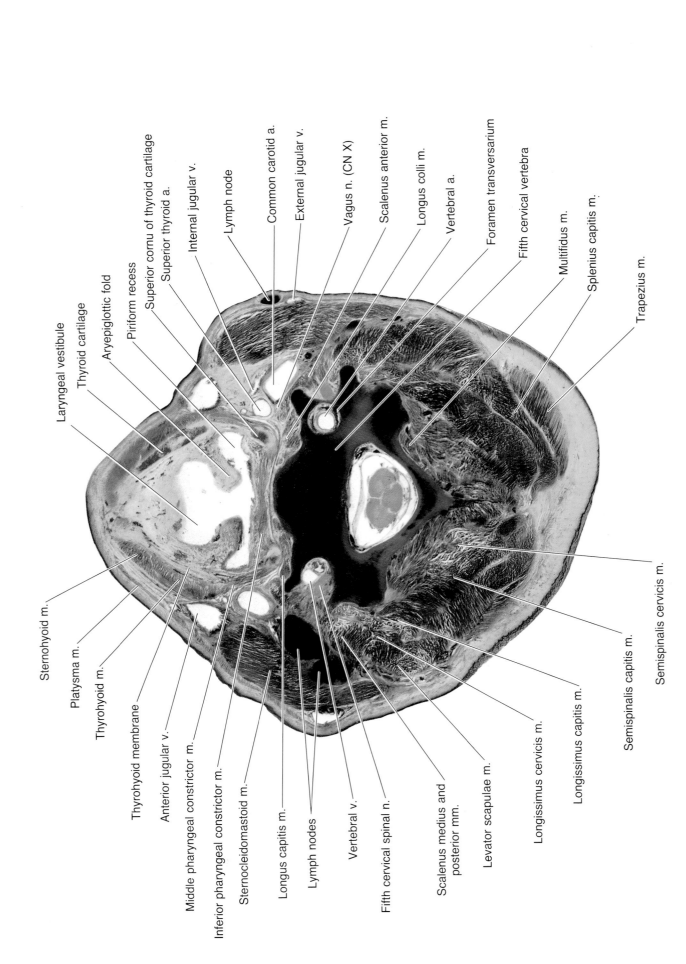

Sternohyoid m.

Platysma m.

Thyrohyoid m.

Thyrohyoid membrane

Anterior jugular v.

Middle pharyngeal constrictor m.

Inferior pharyngeal constrictor m.

Sternocleidomastoid m.

Longus capitis m.

Lymph nodes

Vertebral v.

Fifth cervical spinal n.

Scalenus medius and
posterior mm.

Levator scapulae m.

Longissimus cervicis m.

Longissimus capitis m.

Semispinalis capitis m.

Semispinalis cervicis m.

Laryngeal vestibule

Thyroid cartilage

Aryepiglottic fold

Piriform recess

Superior cornu of thyroid cartilage

Superior thyroid a.

Internal jugular v.

Lymph node

Common carotid a.

External jugular v.

Vagus n. (CN X)

Scalenus anterior m.

Longus colli m.

Vertebral a.

Foramen transversarium

Fifth cervical vertebra

Multifidus m.

Splenius capitis m.

Trapezius m.

The plane of section passes through the thyroid cartilage, laryngeal vestibule, and fifth cervical vertebra. The superior thyroid artery is included in the section.

Transverse Section

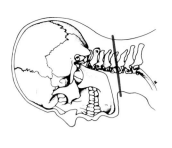

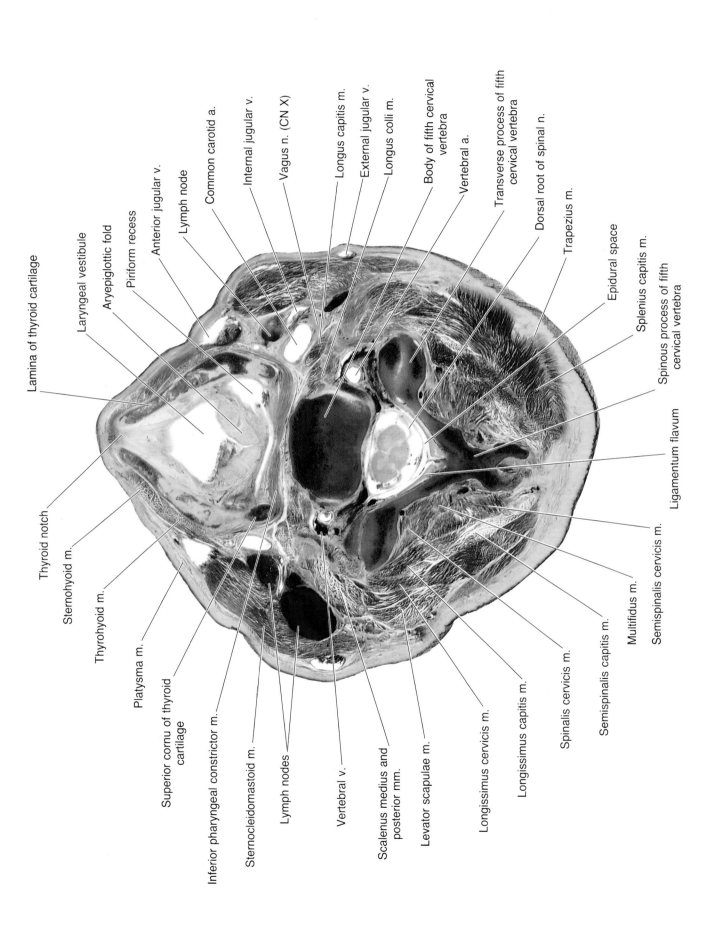

Lamina of thyroid cartilage

Laryngeal vestibule

Aryepiglottic fold

Piriform recess

Anterior jugular v.

Lymph node

Common carotid a.

Internal jugular v.

Vagus n. (CN X)

Longus capitis m.

External jugular v.

Longus colli m.

Body of fifth cervical vertebra

Vertebral a.

Transverse process of fifth cervical vertebra

Dorsal root of spinal n.

Trapezius m.

Epidural space

Splenius capitis m.

Spinous process of fifth cervical vertebra

Thyroid notch

Sternohyoid m.

Thyrohyoid m.

Platysma m.

Superior cornu of thyroid cartilage

Inferior pharyngeal constrictor m.

Sternocleidomastoid m.

Lymph nodes

Vertebral v.

Scalenus medius and posterior mm.

Levator scapulae m.

Longissimus cervicis m.

Longissimus capitis m.

Spinalis cervicis m.

Semispinalis capitis m.

Multifidus m.

Semispinalis cervicis m.

Ligamentum flavum

HEAD AND NECK
Plate 1 – 28

Transverse Section

The plane of section passes through the laminae of the thyroid cartilage, laryngeal vestibule, aryepiglottic fold, and fifth cervical vertebra.

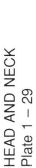

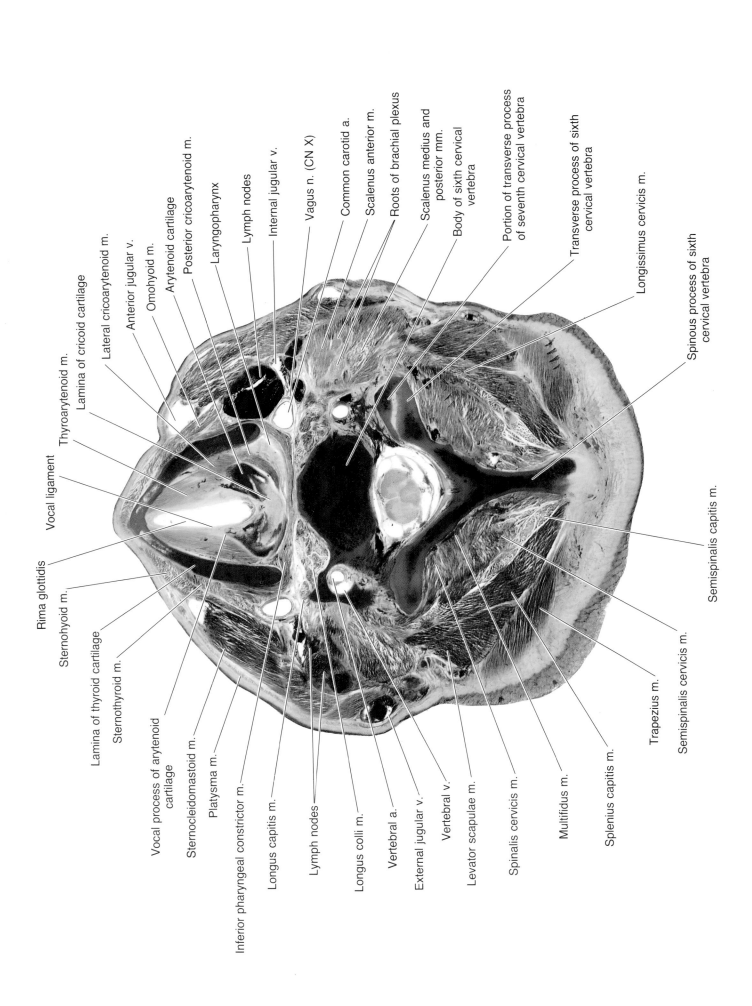

Rima glottidis

Vocal ligament

Thyroarytenoid m.

Lamina of cricoid cartilage

Lateral cricoarytenoid m.

Anterior jugular v.

Omohyoid m.

Arytenoid cartilage

Posterior cricoarytenoid m.

Laryngopharynx

Lymph nodes

Internal jugular v.

Vagus n. (CN X)

Common carotid a.

Scalenus anterior m.

Roots of brachial plexus

Scalenus medius and posterior mm.

Body of sixth cervical vertebra

Portion of transverse process of seventh cervical vertebra

Transverse process of sixth cervical vertebra

Longissimus cervicis m.

Spinous process of sixth cervical vertebra

Semispinalis capitis m.

Sternohyoid m.

Lamina of thyroid cartilage

Sternothyroid m.

Vocal process of arytenoid cartilage

Sternocleidomastoid m.

Platysma m.

Inferior pharyngeal constrictor m.

Longus capitis m.

Lymph nodes

Longus colli m.

Vertebral a.

External jugular v.

Vertebral v.

Levator scapulae m.

Spinalis cervicis m.

Multifidus m.

Splenius capitis m.

Trapezius m.

Semispinalis cervicis m.

The plane of section passes through the thyroid cartilage, rima glottidis, vocal ligaments, and sixth cervical vertebra. Portions of the arytenoid and cricoid cartilages are included in the section.

Transverse Section

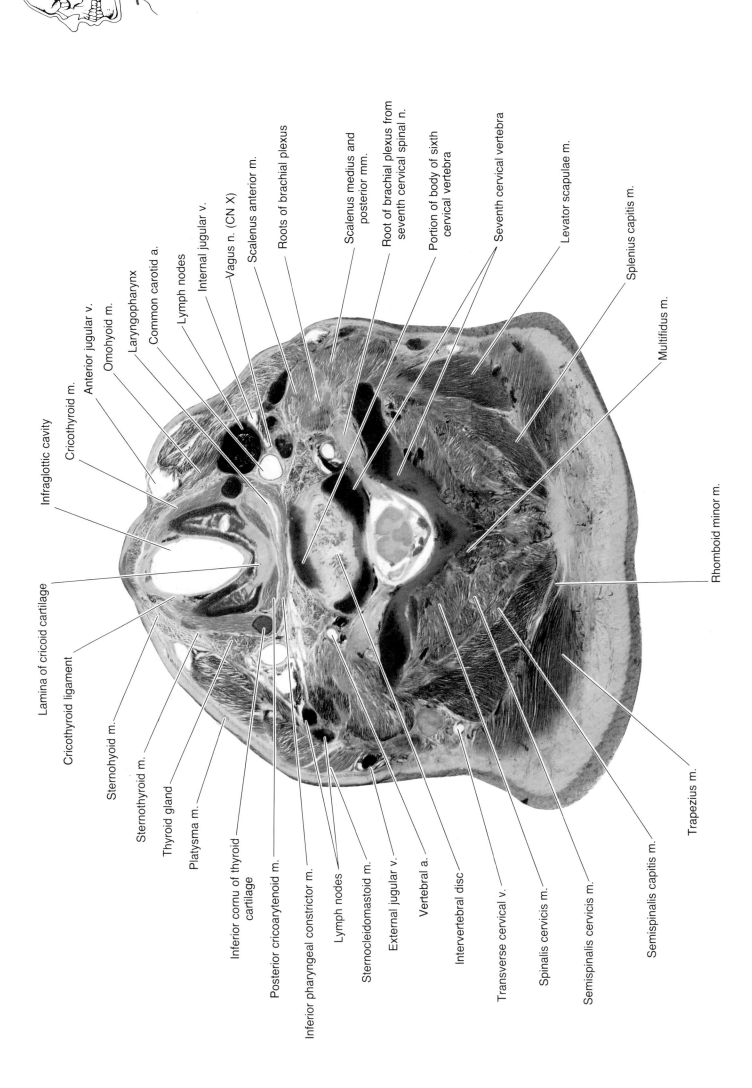

Lamina of cricoid cartilage

Infraglottic cavity

Cricothyroid m.

Anterior jugular v.

Omohyoid m.

Laryngopharynx

Common carotid a.

Lymph nodes

Internal jugular v.

Vagus n. (CN X)

Scalenus anterior m.

Roots of brachial plexus

Scalenus medius and posterior mm.

Root of brachial plexus from seventh cervical spinal n.

Portion of body of sixth cervical vertebra

Seventh cervical vertebra

Levator scapulae m.

Splenius capitis m.

Multifidus m.

Rhomboid minor m.

Trapezius m.

Semispinalis capitis m.

Semispinalis cervicis m.

Spinalis cervicis m.

Transverse cervical v.

Intervertebral disc

Vertebral a.

External jugular v.

Sternocleidomastoid m.

Lymph nodes

Inferior pharyngeal constrictor m.

Posterior cricoarytenoid m.

Inferior cornu of thyroid cartilage

Platysma m.

Thyroid gland

Sternothyroid m.

Sternohyoid m.

Cricothyroid ligament

The plane of section passes through the lamina of the cricoid cartilage, inferior cornu of the thyroid cartilage, and the sixth cervical vertebra.

Transverse Section

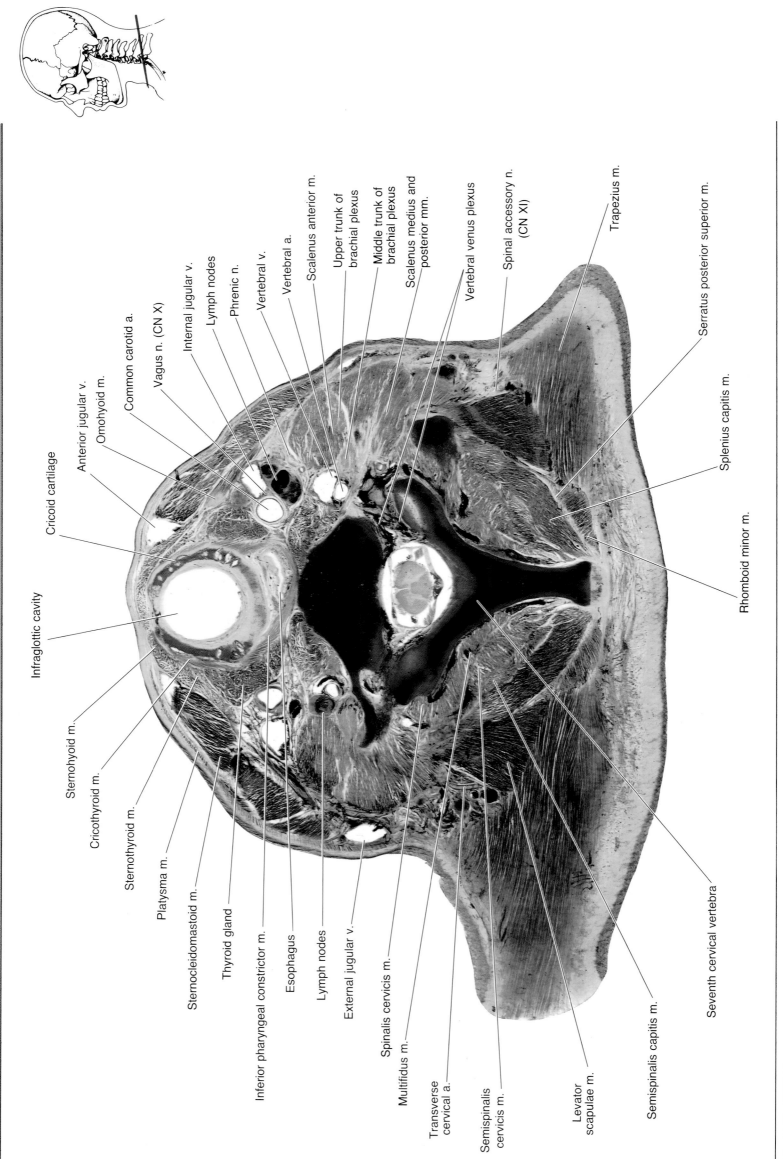

Cricoid cartilage

Infraglottic cavity

Sternohyoid m.

Anterior jugular v.

Omohyoid m.

Common carotid a.

Vagus n. (CN X)

Internal jugular v.

Lymph nodes

Phrenic n.

Vertebral v.

Vertebral a.

Scalenus anterior m.

Upper trunk of brachial plexus

Middle trunk of brachial plexus

Scalenus medius and posterior mm.

Vertebral venus plexus

Spinal accessory n. (CN XI)

Trapezius m.

Serratus posterior superior m.

Splenius capitis m.

Rhomboid minor m.

Cricothyroid m.

Sternothyroid m.

Platysma m.

Sternocleidomastoid m.

Thyroid gland

Inferior pharyngeal constrictor m.

Esophagus

Lymph nodes

External jugular v.

Spinalis cervicis m.

Multifidus m.

Transverse cervical a.

Semispinalis cervicis m.

Levator scapulae m.

Semispinalis capitis m.

Seventh cervical vertebra

HEAD AND NECK
Plate 1 – 31

Transverse Section

The plane of section passes through the cricoid cartilage and seventh cervical vertebra.

Part II

Upper Extremity

Plates 2-1 to 2-25

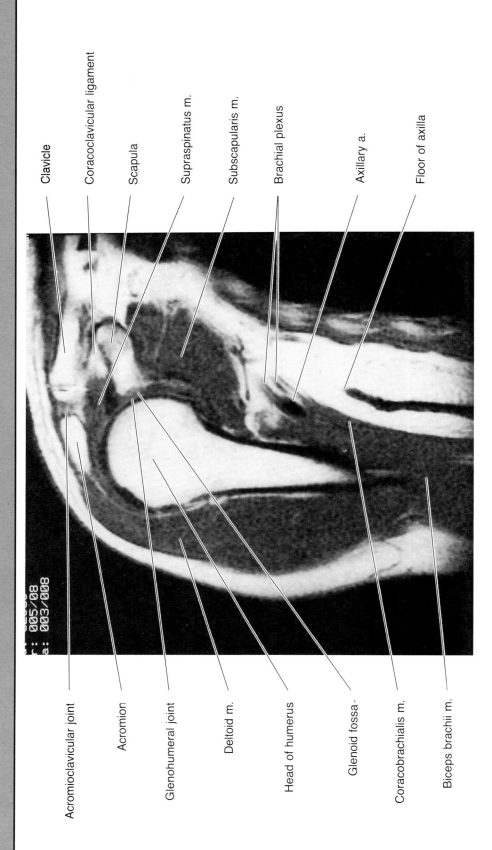

Acromioclavicular joint

Acromion

Glenohumeral joint

Deltoid m.

Head of humerus

Glenoid fossa

Coracobrachialis m.

Biceps brachii m.

Clavicle

Coracoclavicular ligament

Scapula

Supraspinatus m.

Subscapularis m.

Brachial plexus

Axillary a.

Floor of axilla

The sections shown in Plate 2-1 and the accompanying MRI (Plate 2-1 MRI) pass in a coronal plane through the acromioclavicular and glenohumeral joints. The acromioclavicular joint occurs between the acromial process of the scapula and the lateral end of the clavicle. This joint is well displayed in both Plates. However, in Plate 2-1 the trapezoid and conoid portions of the coracoclavicular ligament are well defined as they pass between the distal end of the clavicle and the coracoid process of the scapula. This ligament assists in stabilizing the acromioclavicular joint.

Although the glenohumeral joint can be seen in both Plates, the joint cavity and subscapularis bursa are best seen in Plate 2-1. The glenoid fossa is deepened by the presence of the fibrocartilage rim called the glenoid labrum. The articular surfaces of the head of the humerus and glenoid fossa can be identified in Plate 2-1. The joint capsule and surrounding muscles of the rotator cuff are also best seen in this Plate 2-1. The capsule is reinforced by the glenohumeral ligaments, transverse humeral ligament, and coracohumeral ligament. A portion of coracoacromial ligament can

be seen on the superior aspect of the scapula. All four muscles of the rotator cuff — supraspinatus, infraspinatus, subscapularis, and teres minor — can be identified in Plate 2-1 in association with the capsule of the glenohumeral joint. The stability of the joint is primarily dependent on the tone in the muscles of the rotator cuff.

The axilla can be identified in both Plates. The serratus anterior and the underlying ribs and intercostal muscles can be identified as they form the medial wall of the axilla. Portions of the muscles which form the anterior and posterior walls can also be identified. The pectoralis major and minor muscles contribute to the anterior wall. The subscapularis, latissimus dorsi and teres major muscles form the posterior wall. Within the axilla, the axillary artery, associated cords of the brachial plexus, and lymph nodes can be identified. In Plate 2-1, the musculocutaneous nerve can be seen running downward and laterally as it pierces the coracobrachialis muscle. Near the apex of the axilla the long thoracic nerve can be identified as it passes along the surface of the serratus anterior muscle.

Plate 2-1 MRI
Coronal Section

Coracoclavicular (trapezoid) ligament
Trapezius m.
Coracoclavicular (conoid) ligament
Scapula
Omohyoid m.
Long thoracic n.
Glenoid fossa
Serratus anterior m.
Subscapularis m.
Lateral cord of brachial plexus
Posterior cord of brachial plexus
Medial cord of brachial plexus
Subscapular a.
Thoracodorsal n.
Axillary lymph node
Axillary v.
Axillary a.
Radial n.
Musculocutaneous n.
Coracobrachialis m.
Floor of axilla
Intercostal m.
Biceps brachii m.

Coracoacromial ligament
Clavicle
Acromioclavicular joint
Acromion
Subacromial bursa
Supraspinatus m.
Infraspinatus m.
Cavity of glenohumeral joint
Glenoid labrum
Head of humerus
Deltoid m.
Epiphyseal line
Teres minor m.
Surgical neck of humerus
Subscapularis bursa
Axillary n.
Posterior humeral circumflex v.
Posterior humeral circumflex a.
Latissimus dorsi tendon
Teres major m.
Lateral head of triceps m.

Section of the shoulder through the anterior portion of the articulation of the head of the humerus with the glenoid fossa. The acromioclavicular joint and coracoclavicular ligament are included.

Coronal Section

UPPER EXTREMITY.
Plate 2-1

Transverse Section

Capsule of sternoclavicular joint

Head of clavicle

Pectoralis major m.

First rib

Upper lobe of right lung

Intercostal m.

Subscapularis m.

Serratus anterior m.

Supraspinatus m.

Rhomboid major m.

Rhomboid minor m.

Levator scapulae m.

Trapezius m.

Axillary a.

Deltoid branch of thoracoacromial a.

Cords of brachial plexus

Cephalic v.

Pectoralis minor m.

Coracoid process of scapula

Subscapularis tendon

Long head of biceps brachii tendon

Deltoid m.

Greater tubercle

Intertubecular sulcus (Bicipital groove)

Lesser tubercle

Head of humerus

Cavity of glenohumeral joint

Articular cartilage

Teres minor m.

Supraspinatus tendon

Glenoid fossa

Scapula

Infraspinatus m.

Spine of scapula

UPPER EXTREMITY.
Plate 2-2

Section of the shoulder through the articulation of the head of the humerus with the glenoid fossa.
The axillary artery and cords of the brachial plexus can be seen at the lateral border of the 1st rib.

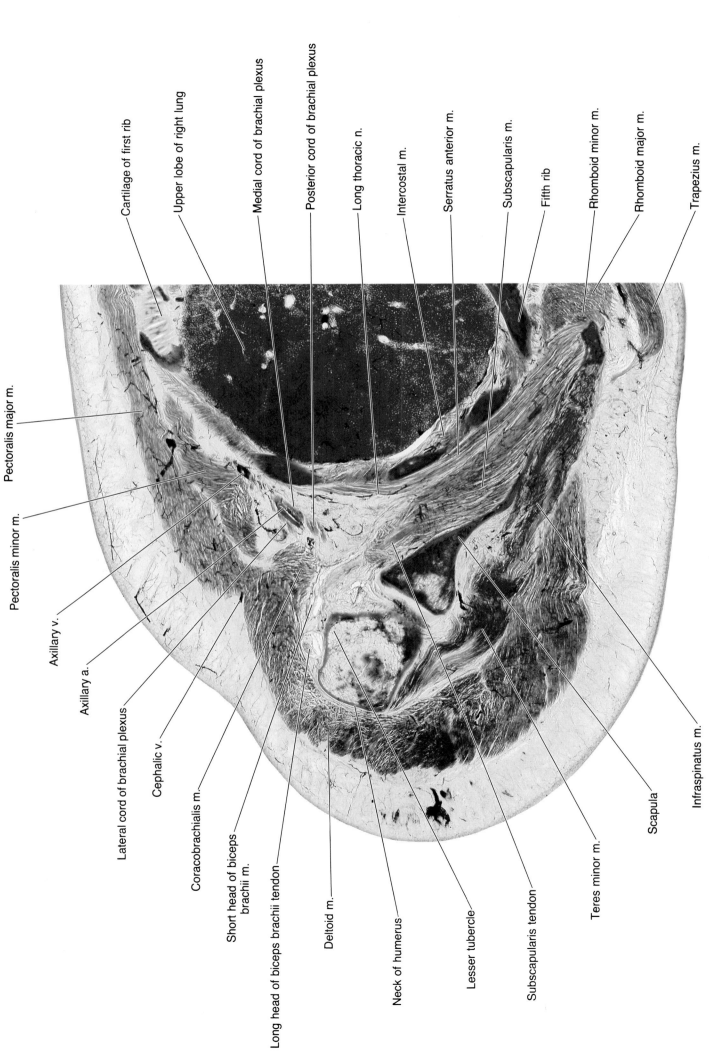

Pectoralis major m.

Pectoralis minor m.

Axillary v.

Axillary a.

Lateral cord of brachial plexus

Cephalic v.

Coracobrachialis m.

Short head of biceps brachii m.

Long head of biceps brachii tendon

Deltoid m.

Neck of humerus

Lesser tubercle

Subscapularis tendon

Teres minor m.

Scapula

Infraspinatus m.

Cartilage of first rib

Upper lobe of right lung

Medial cord of brachial plexus

Posterior cord of brachial plexus

Long thoracic n.

Intercostal m.

Serratus anterior m.

Subscapularis m.

Fifth rib

Rhomboid minor m.

Rhomboid major m.

Trapezius m.

Transverse Section

Section of the shoulder through the neck of the humerus. The medial, lateral, and posterior cords of the brachial plexus can be seen in association with the axillary artery near the apex of the axilla.

UPPER EXTREMITY.
Plate 2-3

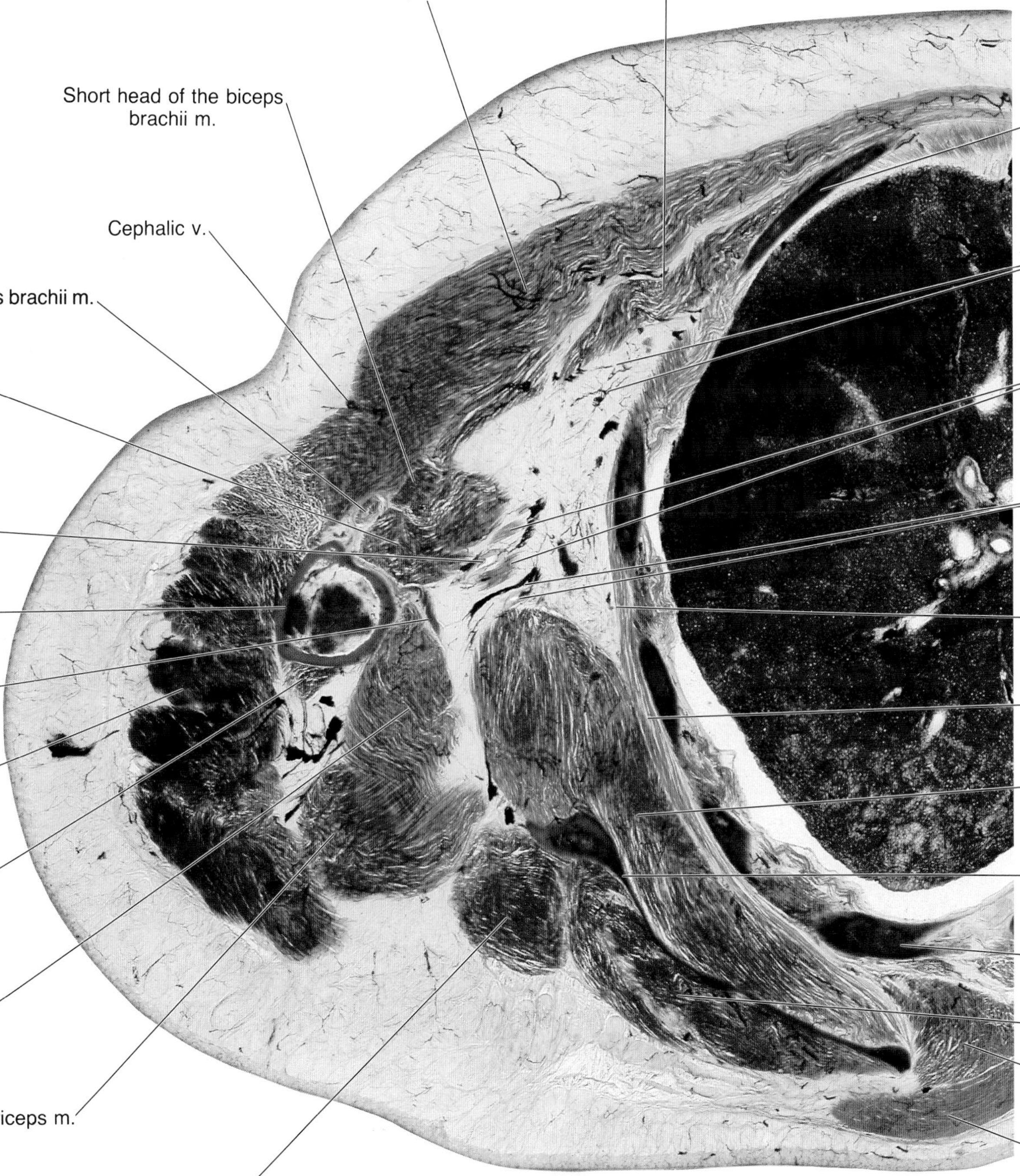

Pectoralis minor m.

Pectoralis major m.

Short head of the biceps brachii m.

Cephalic v.

Long head of biceps brachii m.

Coracobrachialis m.

Axillary a.

Shaft of humerus

Latissimus dorsi tendon

Deltoid m.

Lateral head of triceps m.

Teres major m.

Long head of triceps m.

Second rib

Lateral thoracic a. & v.

Branches of brachial plexus

Subscapular a. & v.

Long thoracic n.

Serratus anterior m.

Subscapularis m.

Scapula

Sixth rib

Infraspinatus m.

Rhomboid major m.

Trapezius m.

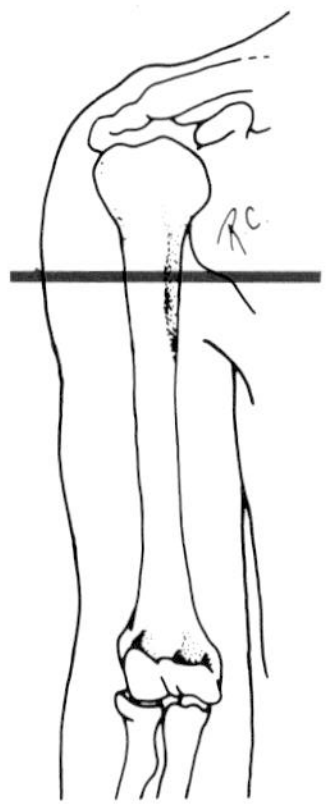

Teres minor m.

Transverse Section

UPPER EXTREMITY.
Plate 2-4

Section through the axilla at the proximal end of the lateral head of the Triceps and just inferior to the insertion of the Latissimus dorsi and Teres major into the medial lip of the bicipital groove.

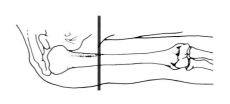

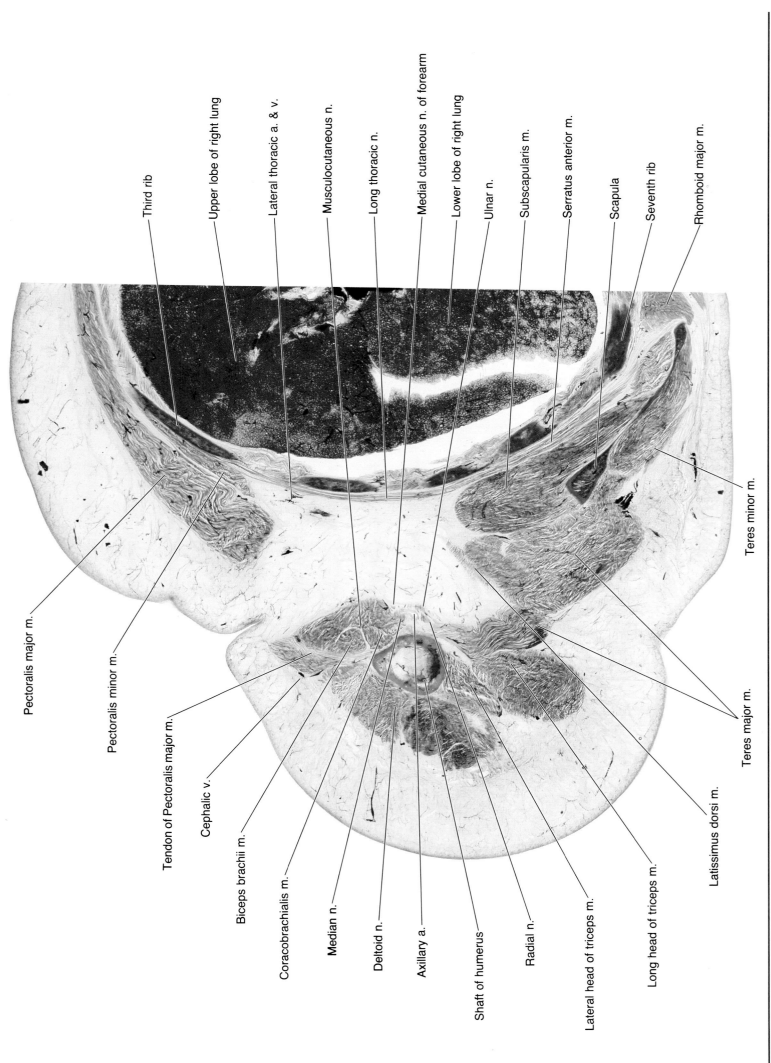

Third rib

Upper lobe of right lung

Lateral thoracic a. & v.

Musculocutaneous n.

Long thoracic n.

Medial cutaneous n. of forearm

Lower lobe of right lung

Ulnar n.

Subscapularis m.

Serratus anterior m.

Scapula

Seventh rib

Rhomboid major m.

Pectoralis major m.

Pectoralis minor m.

Tendon of Pectoralis major m.

Cephalic v.

Biceps brachii m.

Coracobrachialis m.

Median n.

Deltoid n.

Axillary a.

Shaft of humerus

Radial n.

Lateral head of triceps m.

Long head of triceps m.

Latissimus dorsi m.

Teres major m.

Teres minor m.

UPPER EXTREMITY.
Plate 2-5

Section through the floor of the axilla at the distal end of the insertion of the Pectoralis major into the lateral lip of the bicipital groove and proximal to the insertion of the Coracobrachialis.

Transverse Section

Biceps brachii m.

Musculocutaneous n.

Brachial fascia

Brachial a.

Median n.

Medial cutaneous n. of forearm

Basilic v.

Ulnar n.

Medial head of triceps brachii m.

Cephalic v.

Long head of triceps brachii m.

Brachialis m.

Deltoid tuberosity

Deltoid m.

Shaft of humerus

Radial n.

Profunda brachii a. & v.

Lateral head of triceps brachii m.

UPPER EXTREMITY.
Plate 2-6

Section of the arm through the deltoid tuberosity and proximal end of the origin of the Brachialis.
The insertion of the Coracobrachialis is just proximal to this level.

Transverse Section

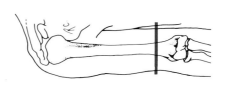

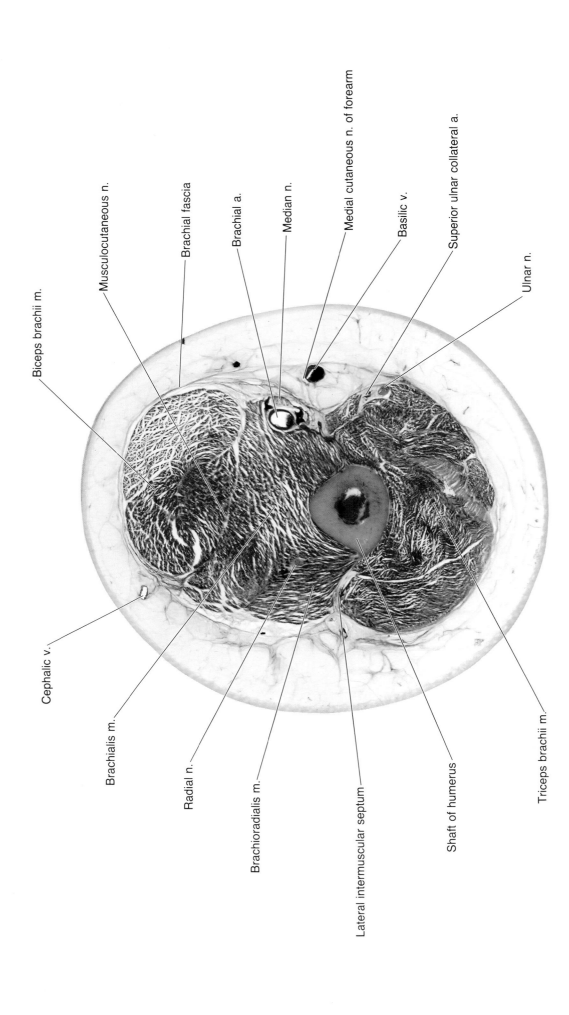

Biceps brachii m.

Musculocutaneous n.

Brachial fascia

Brachial a.

Median n.

Medial cutaneous n. of forearm

Basilic v.

Superior ulnar collateral a.

Ulnar n.

Cephalic v.

Brachialis m.

Radial n.

Brachioradialis m.

Lateral intermuscular septum

Shaft of humerus

Triceps brachii m.

Transverse Section

Section of the arm just proximal to the supracondylar ridges. The ulnar nerve is located in the posterior compartment; the radial nerve, in the anterior compartment deep to the Brachioradialis.

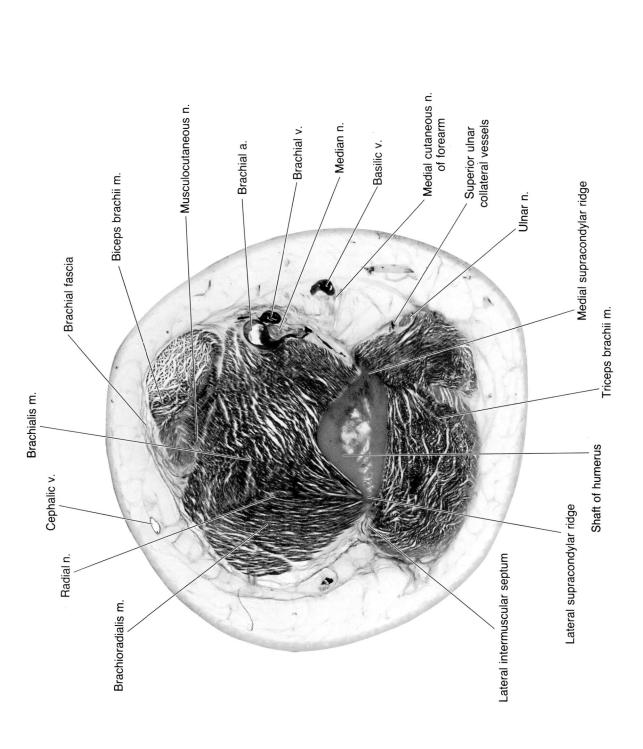

Musculocutaneous n.

Brachial a.

Brachial v.

Median n.

Basilic v.

Medial cutaneous n. of forearm

Superior ulnar collateral vessels

Ulnar n.

Biceps brachii m.

Brachial fascia

Brachialis m.

Cephalic v.

Radial n.

Brachioradialis m.

Medial supracondylar ridge

Triceps brachii m.

Shaft of humerus

Lateral supracondylar ridge

Lateral intermuscular septum

UPPER EXTREMITY.
Plate 2-8

Transverse Section

Section of the arm through the proximal end of the supracondylar ridges.

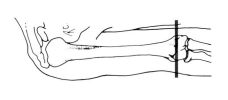

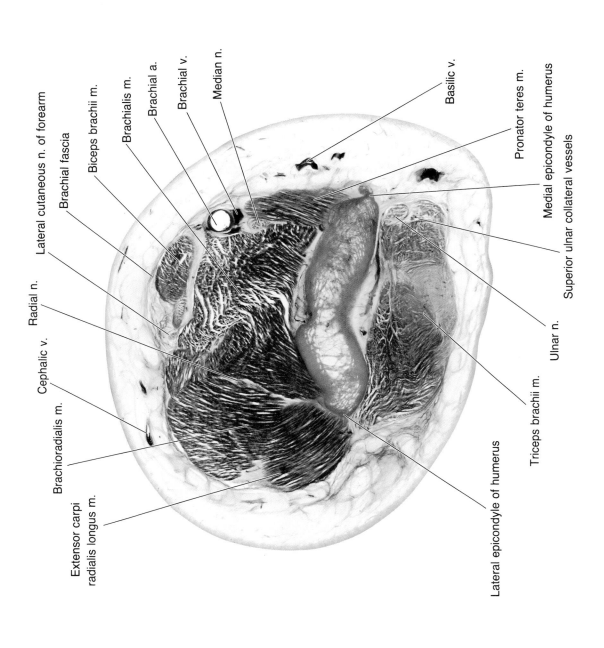

Lateral cutaneous n. of forearm

Brachial fascia

Biceps brachii m.

Brachialis m.

Brachial a.

Brachial v.

Median n.

Basilic v.

Radial n.

Cephalic v.

Brachioradialis m.

Extensor carpi
radialis longus m.

Lateral epicondyle of humerus

Triceps brachii m.

Ulnar n.

Pronator teres m.

Medial epicondyle of humerus

Superior ulnar collateral vessels

Transverse Section

Section of the arm through the epicondyles.
The ulnar nerve lies posterior to the medial epicondyle.

UPPER EXTREMITY.
Plate 2-9

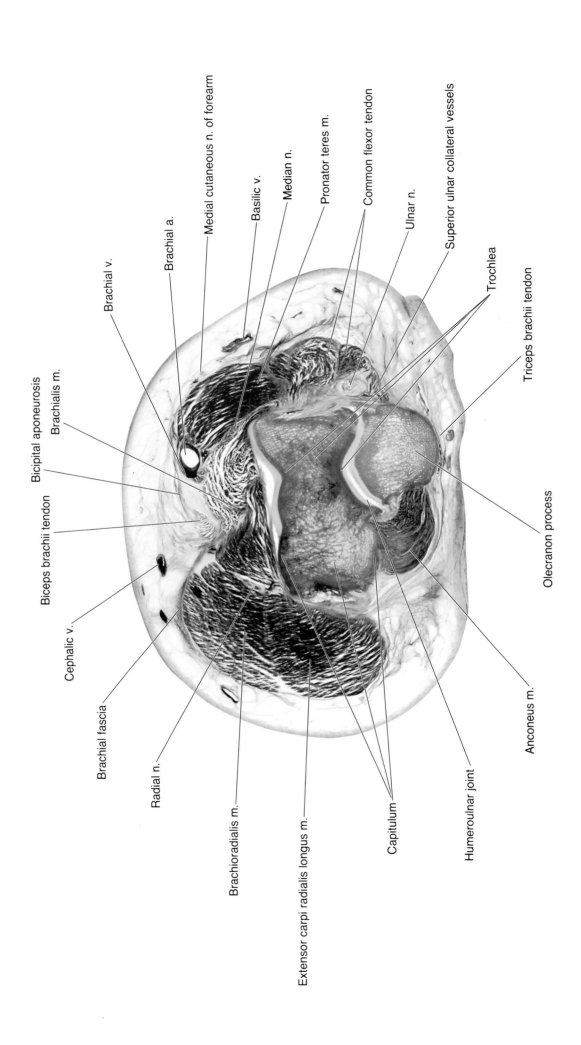

Medial cutaneous n. of forearm

Basilic v.

Median n.

Pronator teres m.

Common flexor tendon

Ulnar n.

Superior ulnar collateral vessels

Trochlea

Triceps brachii tendon

Brachial a.

Brachial v.

Bicipital aponeurosis

Brachialis m.

Biceps brachii tendon

Cephalic v.

Brachial fascia

Radial n.

Brachioradialis m.

Extensor carpi radialis longus m.

Capitulum

Humeroulnar joint

Anconeus m.

Olecranon process

Transverse Section

Section of the arm through humeroulnar joint. Portions of capitulum and trochlea of the humerus and the olecranon process of the ulna are included in the section.

UPPER EXTREMITY.
Plate 2-10

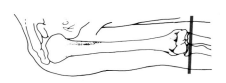

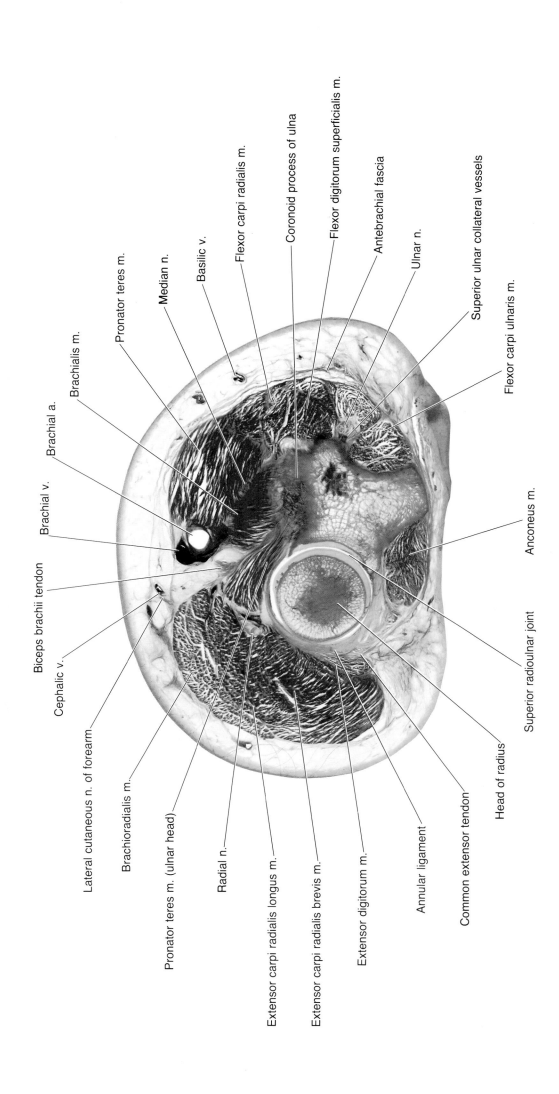

Brachialis m.

Pronator teres m.

Median n.

Basilic v.

Flexor carpi radialis m.

Coronoid process of ulna

Flexor digitorum superficialis m.

Antebrachial fascia

Ulnar n.

Superior ulnar collateral vessels

Flexor carpi ulnaris m.

Brachial a.

Brachial v.

Biceps brachii tendon

Cephalic v.

Lateral cutaneous n. of forearm

Brachioradialis m.

Pronator teres m. (ulnar head)

Radial n.

Extensor carpi radialis longus m.

Extensor carpi radialis brevis m.

Extensor digitorum m.

Annular ligament

Common extensor tendon

Head of radius

Superior radioulnar joint

Anconeus m.

UPPER EXTREMITY.
Plate 2-11

Section of the forearm through proximal radioulnar joint. The head of the radius and coronoid
process of the ulna (the attachment site of the Brachialis) are included in the section.

Transverse Section

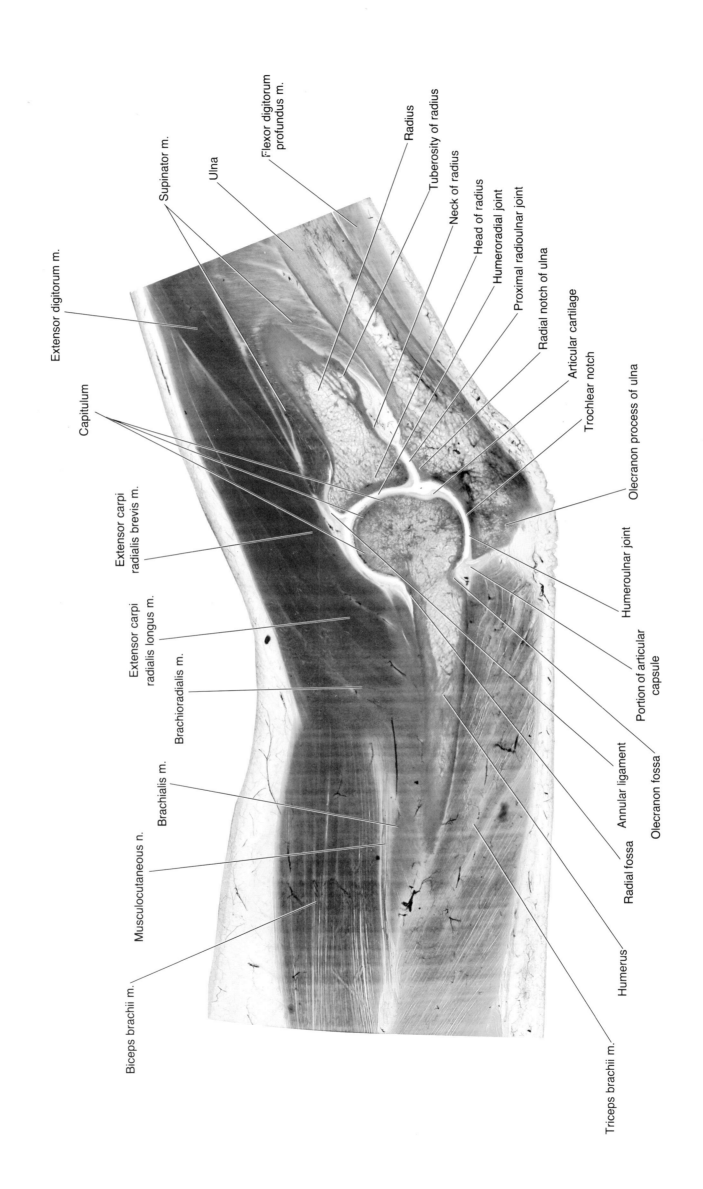

Section passing obliquely through the elbow and including the capitulum of the humerus, the head
and tuberosity of the radius, and portions of the shaft and olecranon process of the ulna.

Longitudinal Section

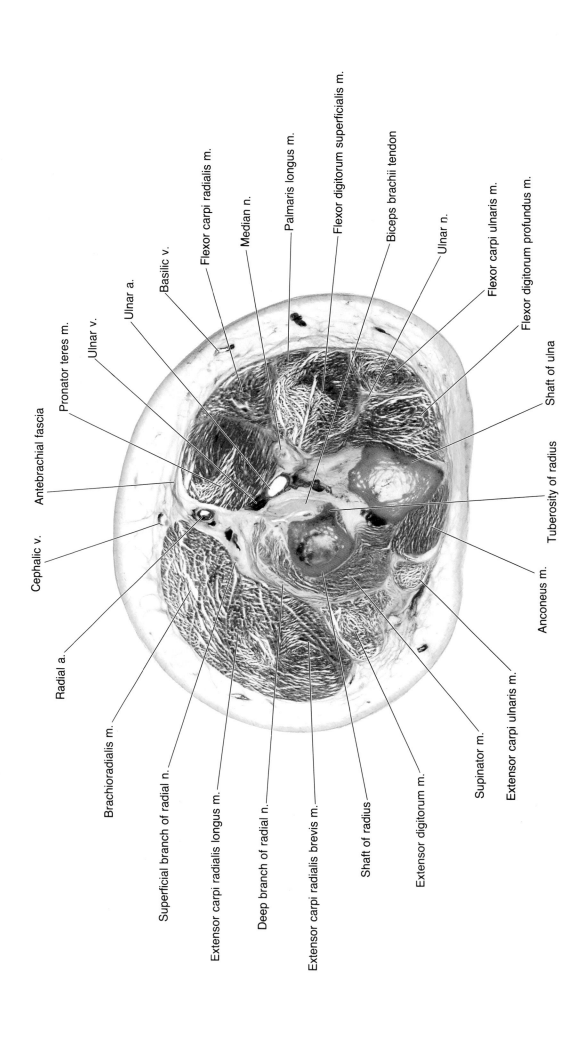

Cephalic v.

Antebrachial fascia

Radial a.

Pronator teres m.

Ulnar v.

Ulnar a.

Basilic v.

Flexor carpi radialis m.

Median n.

Palmaris longus m.

Flexor digitorum superficialis m.

Biceps brachii tendon

Ulnar n.

Flexor carpi ulnaris m.

Flexor digitorum profundus m.

Shaft of ulna

Tuberosity of radius

Anconeus m.

Extensor carpi ulnaris m.

Supinator m.

Extensor digitorum m.

Shaft of radius

Extensor carpi radialis brevis m.

Deep branch of radial n.

Extensor carpi radialis longus m.

Superficial branch of radial n.

Brachioradialis m.

UPPER EXTREMITY.
Plate 2-13

Section of the forearm through the tuberosity of the radius (attachment site of the Biceps brachii tendon) and shaft of the ulna. The Supinator can be seen as it passes from the ulna to the radius.

Transverse Section

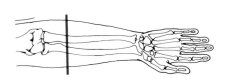

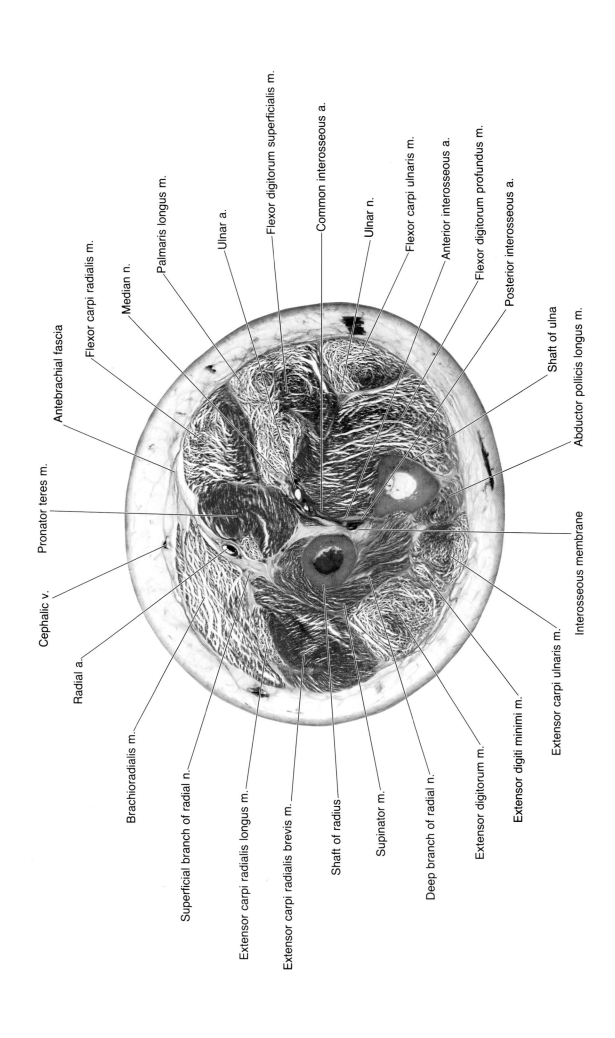

Flexor digitorum superficialis m.

Common interosseous a.

Palmaris longus m.

Ulnar a.

Ulnar n.

Median n.

Flexor carpi ulnaris m.

Flexor carpi radialis m.

Anterior interosseous a.

Antebrachial fascia

Flexor digitorum profundus m.

Posterior interosseous a.

Pronator teres m.

Shaft of ulna

Cephalic v.

Abductor pollicis longus m.

Radial a.

Brachioradialis m.

Interosseous membrane

Superficial branch of radial n.

Extensor carpi ulnaris m.

Extensor carpi radialis longus m.

Extensor digiti minimi m.

Extensor carpi radialis brevis m.

Extensor digitorum m.

Shaft of radius

Deep branch of radial n.

Supinator m.

UPPER EXTREMITY.
Plate 2-14

Transverse Section

Section of the forearm just distal to the tuberosity of the radius. The common interosseous artery
and its anterior and posterior branches are included in the section.

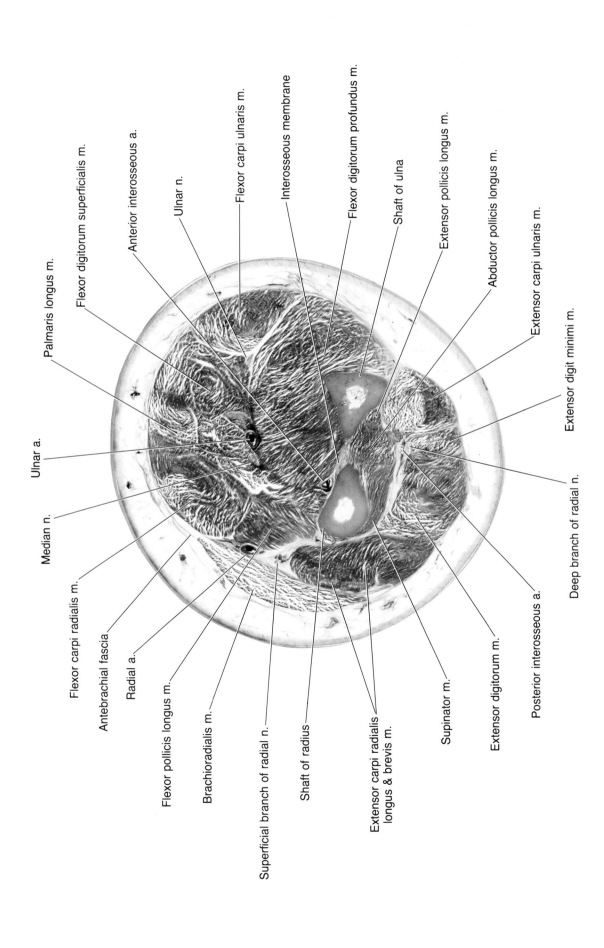

Palmaris longus m.

Flexor digitorum superficialis m.

Anterior interosseous a.

Ulnar n.

Flexor carpi ulnaris m.

Interosseous membrane

Flexor digitorum profundus m.

Shaft of ulna

Extensor pollicis longus m.

Abductor pollicis longus m.

Extensor carpi ulnaris m.

Extensor digit minimi m.

Ulnar a.

Median n.

Flexor carpi radialis m.

Antebrachial fascia

Radial a.

Flexor pollicis longus m.

Brachioradialis m.

Superficial branch of radial n.

Shaft of radius

Extensor carpi radialis
longus & brevis m.

Supinator m.

Extensor digitorum m.

Posterior interosseous a.

Deep branch of radial n.

UPPER EXTREMITY.
Plate 2-15

Section of the forearm at the distal end of the Supinator. In the posterior compartment, proximal portions of the Adductor pollicis longus and Extensor pollicis longus are included in the section.

Transverse Section

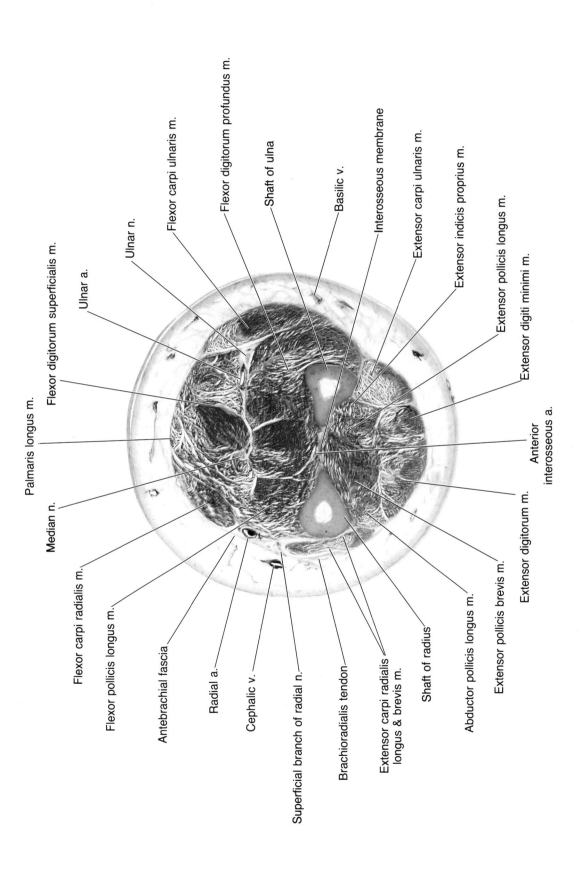

Palmaris longus m.

Flexor digitorum superficialis m.

Ulnar a.

Ulnar n.

Flexor carpi ulnaris m.

Flexor digitorum profundus m.

Shaft of ulna

Basilic v.

Interosseous membrane

Extensor carpi ulnaris m.

Extensor indicis proprius m.

Extensor pollicis longus m.

Extensor digiti minimi m.

Median n.

Flexor carpi radialis m.

Flexor pollicis longus m.

Antebrachial fascia

Radial a.

Cephalic v.

Superficial branch of radial n.

Brachioradialis tendon

Extensor carpi radialis
longus & brevis m.

Shaft of radius

Abductor pollicis longus m.

Extensor pollicis brevis m.

Extensor digitorum m.

Anterior
interosseous a.

Section of the forearm at its distal third. The separate slips of the Flexor and Extensor digitorum muscles are evident at this level.

Transverse Section

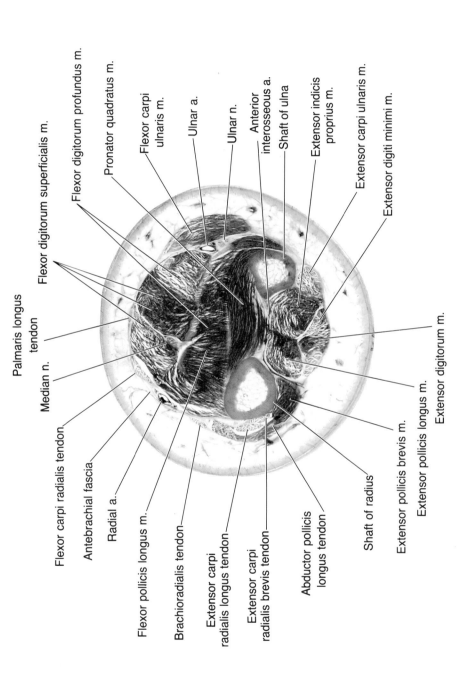

Flexor digitorum profundus m.

Pronator quadratus m.

Flexor carpi ulnaris m.

Ulnar a.

Ulnar n.

Anterior interosseous a.

Shaft of ulna

Extensor indicis proprius m.

Extensor carpi ulnaris m.

Extensor digiti minimi m.

Flexor digitorum superficialis m.

Palmaris longus tendon

Median n.

Antebrachial fascia

Radial a.

Flexor pollicis longus m.

Brachioradialis tendon

Extensor carpi radialis longus tendon

Extensor carpi radialis brevis tendon

Abductor pollicis longus tendon

Shaft of radius

Extensor pollicis brevis m.

Extensor pollicis longus m.

Extensor digitorum m.

Flexor carpi radialis tendon

Section of the forearm at the proximal border of the Pronator quadratus. On the radial side, the Extensor carpi radialis longus and brevis tendons lie deep to the Abductor pollicis longus tendon.

Transverse Section

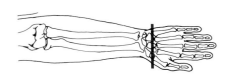

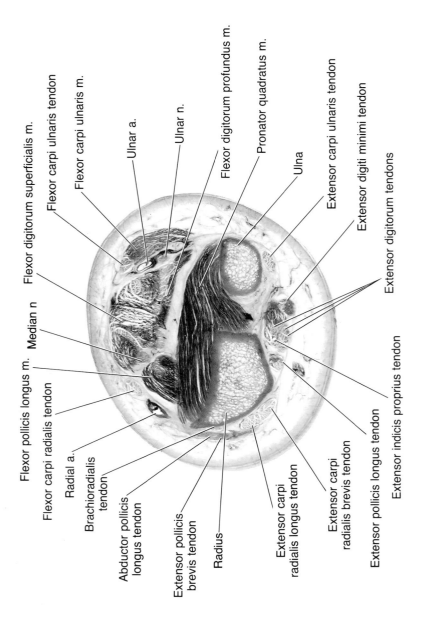

Flexor pollicis longus m.

Flexor digitorum superficialis m.

Flexor carpi ulnaris tendon

Flexor carpi ulnaris m.

Ulnar a.

Ulnar n.

Flexor digitorum profundus m.

Pronator quadratus m.

Ulna

Extensor carpi ulnaris tendon

Extensor digiti minimi tendon

Extensor digitorum tendons

Median n

Abductor pollicis longus tendon

Flexor carpi radialis tendon

Radial a.

Brachioradialis tendon

Extensor pollicis brevis tendon

Radius

Extensor carpi radialis longus tendon

Extensor carpi radialis brevis tendon

Extensor pollicis longus tendon

Extensor indicis proprius tendon

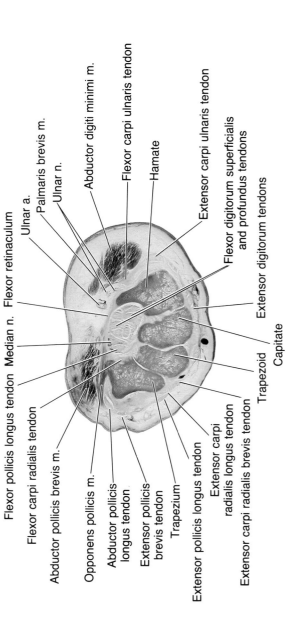

Flexor pollicis longus tendon

Median n.

Flexor retinaculum

Ulnar a.

Palmaris brevis m.

Ulnar n.

Abductor digiti minimi m.

Flexor carpi ulnaris tendon

Hamate

Extensor carpi ulnaris tendon

Flexor digitorum superficialis and profundus tendons

Extensor digitorum tendons

Flexor carpi radialis tendon

Abductor pollicis brevis m.

Opponens pollicis m.

Abductor pollicis longus tendon

Extensor pollicis brevis tendon

Trapezium

Extensor pollicis longus tendon

Extensor carpi radialis longus tendon

Extensor carpi radialis brevis tendon

Trapezoid

Capitate

Plate 2-18:   Section of the forearm just proximal to the wrist at the distal border of the Pronator quadratus.
Plate 2-19:   Transverse section through the wrist at the distal row of carpal bones (carpal tunnel).

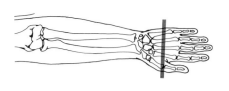

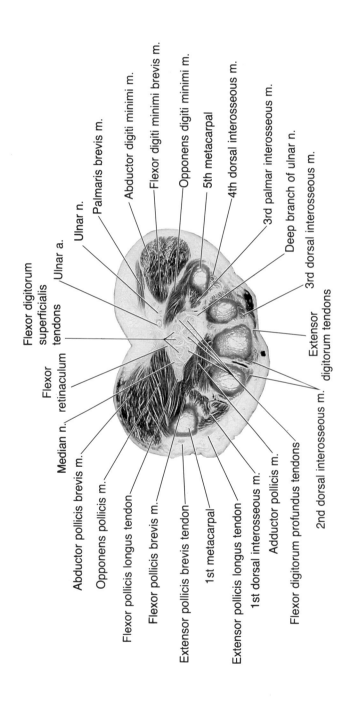

Flexor digitorum
superficialis
tendons

Flexor
retinaculum

Ulnar a.

Ulnar n.

Palmaris brevis m.

Abductor digiti minimi m.

Flexor digiti minimi brevis m.

Opponens digiti minimi m.

5th metacarpal

4th dorsal interosseous m.

3rd palmar interosseous m.

Deep branch of ulnar n.

3rd dorsal interosseous m.

Extensor
digitorum tendons

Median n.

Abductor pollicis brevis m.

Opponens pollicis m.

Flexor pollicis longus tendon

Flexor pollicis brevis m.

Extensor pollicis brevis tendon

1st metacarpal

Extensor pollicis longus tendon

1st dorsal interosseous m.

Adductor pollicis m.

Flexor digitorum profundus tendons

2nd dorsal interosseous m.

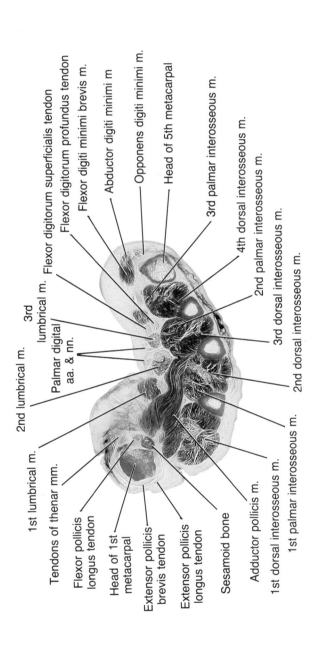

2nd lumbrical m.

3rd
lumbrical m.

Flexor digitorum superficialis tendon

Flexor digitorum profundus tendon

Flexor digiti minimi brevis m.

Abductor digiti minimi m

Opponens digiti minimi m.

Head of 5th metacarpal

3rd palmar interosseous m.

4th dorsal interosseous m.

2nd palmar interosseous m.

3rd dorsal interosseous m.

2nd dorsal interosseous m.

1st lumbrical m.

Tendons of thenar mm.

Flexor pollicis
longus tendon

Head of 1st
metacarpal

Extensor pollicis
brevis tendon

Extensor pollicis
longus tendon

Sesamoid bone

Adductor pollicis m.

1st dorsal interosseous m.

1st palmar interosseous m.

Palmar digital
aa. & nn.

Plate 2-20: Transverse section through the hand at the proximal end of the metacarpal bones.
Plate 2-21: Transverse section through the hand at the distal end of the metacarpal bones.

Transverse Sections

UPPER EXTREMITY.
Plates 2-20 and 2-21

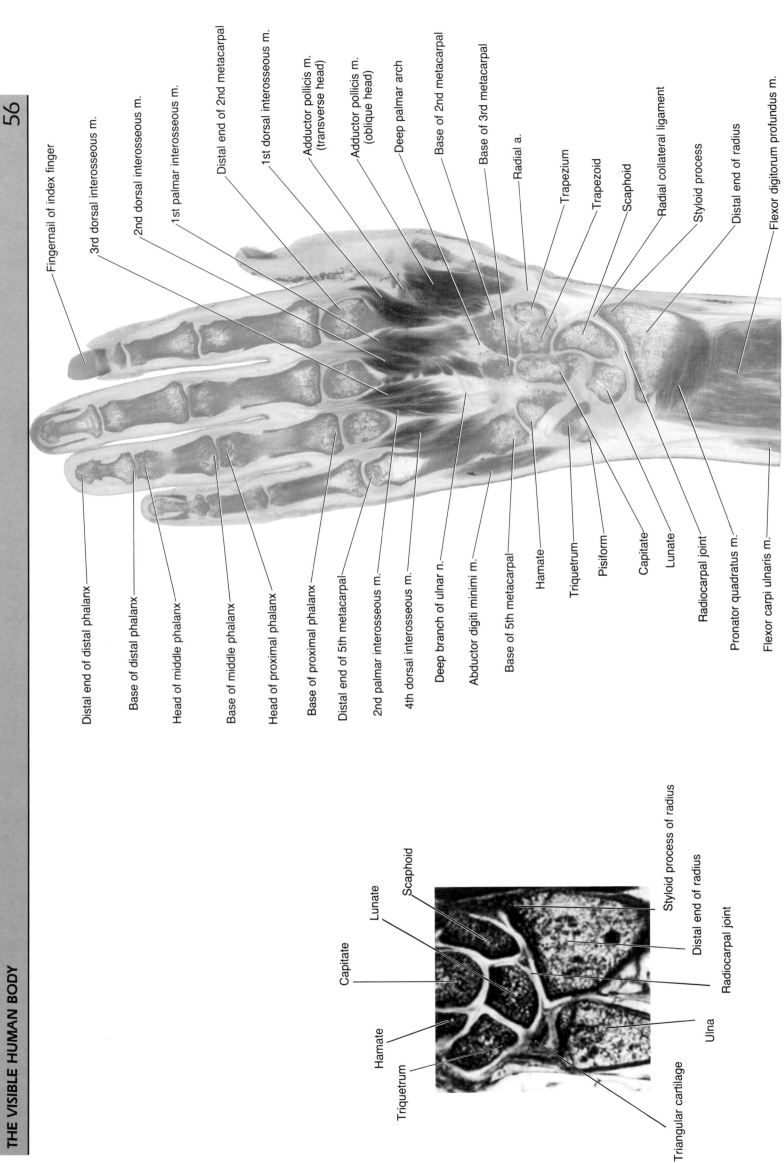

Fingernail of index finger

3rd dorsal interosseous m.

2nd dorsal interosseous m.

1st palmar interosseous m.

Distal end of 2nd metacarpal

1st dorsal interosseous m.

Adductor pollicis m. (transverse head)

Adductor pollicis m. (oblique head)

Deep palmar arch

Base of 2nd metacarpal

Base of 3rd metacarpal

Radial a.

Trapezium

Trapezoid

Scaphoid

Radial collateral ligament

Styloid process

Distal end of radius

Flexor digitorum profundus m.

Distal end of distal phalanx

Base of distal phalanx

Head of middle phalanx

Base of middle phalanx

Head of proximal phalanx

Base of proximal phalanx

Distal end of 5th metacarpal

2nd palmar interosseous m.

4th dorsal interosseous m.

Deep branch of ulnar n.

Abductor digiti minimi m.

Base of 5th metacarpal

Hamate

Triquetrum

Pisiform

Capitate

Lunate

Radiocarpal joint

Pronator quadratus m.

Flexor carpi ulnaris m.

Capitate

Lunate

Scaphoid

Hamate

Triquetrum

Triangular cartilage

Styloid process of radius

Distal end of radius

Radiocarpal joint

Ulna

Section of the dorsal aspect of the hand passing through the interosseous muscles. Portions of all carpal bones, deep palmar arch, and deep branch of the ulnar nerve are included in the section.

Coronal Section
Dorsal View of Left Hand

UPPER EXTREMITY.
Plate 2-22

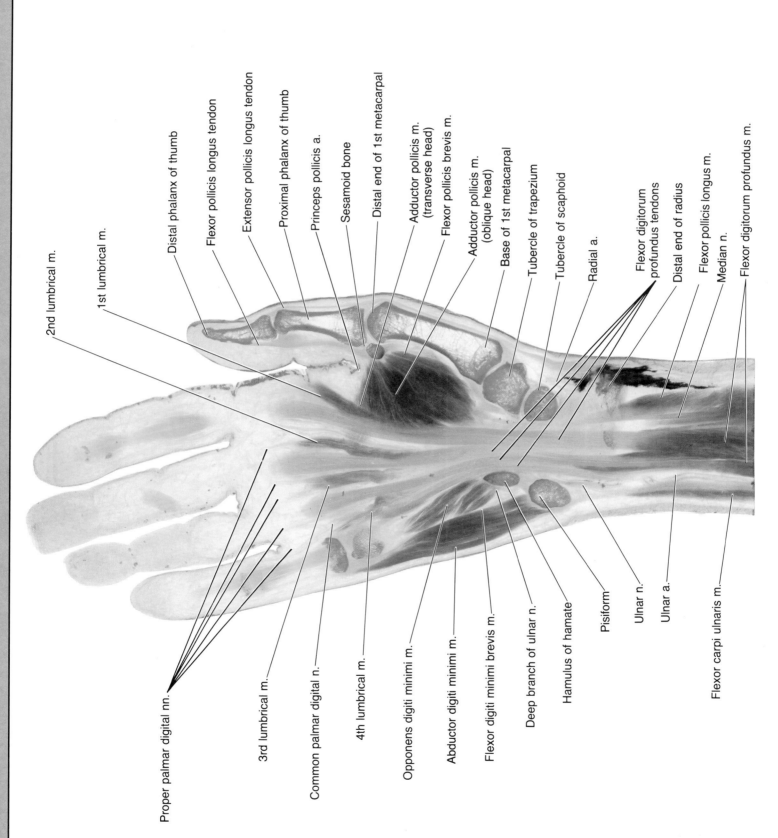

2nd lumbrical m.

1st lumbrical m.

Distal phalanx of thumb

Flexor pollicis longus tendon

Extensor pollicis longus tendon

Proximal phalanx of thumb

Princeps pollicis a.

Sesamoid bone

Distal end of 1st metacarpal

Adductor pollicis m. (transverse head)

Flexor pollicis brevis m.

Adductor pollicis m. (oblique head)

Base of 1st metacarpal

Tubercle of trapezium

Tubercle of scaphoid

Radial a.

Flexor digitorum profundus tendons

Distal end of radius

Flexor pollicis longus m.

Median n.

Flexor digitorum profundus m.

Proper palmar digital nn.

3rd lumbrical m.

Common palmar digital n.

4th lumbrical m.

Opponens digiti minimi m.

Abductor digiti minimi m.

Flexor digiti minimi brevis m.

Deep branch of ulnar n.

Hamulus of hamate

Pisiform

Ulnar n.

Ulnar a.

Flexor carpi ulnaris m.

UPPER EXTREMITY.
Plate 2-23

Section of the hand passing longitudinally through the carpal tunnel. Portions of the hamate, pisiform, trapezium, scaphoid and Flexor digitorum profundus tendons are included in the section.

Coronal Section
Dorsal View of Left Hand

Part III

Thorax

Plates 3-1 to 3-14

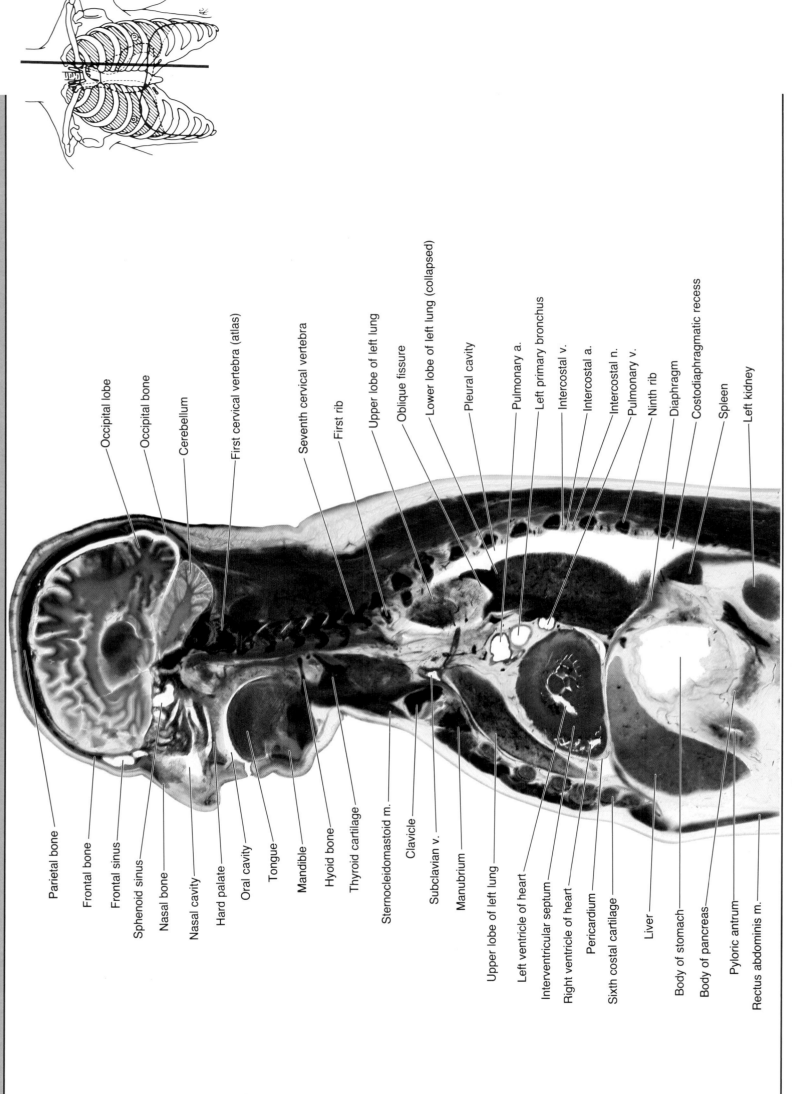

Parietal bone
Frontal bone
Frontal sinus
Sphenoid sinus
Nasal bone
Nasal cavity
Hard palate
Oral cavity
Tongue
Mandible
Hyoid bone
Thyroid cartilage
Sternocleidomastoid m.
Clavicle
Subclavian v.
Manubrium
Upper lobe of left lung
Left ventricle of heart
Interventricular septum
Right ventricle of heart
Pericardium
Sixth costal cartilage
Liver
Body of stomach
Body of pancreas
Pyloric antrum
Rectus abdominis m.

Occipital lobe
Occipital bone
Cerebellum
First cervical vertebra (atlas)
Seventh cervical vertebra
First rib
Upper lobe of left lung
Oblique fissure
Lower lobe of left lung (collapsed)
Pleural cavity
Pulmonary a.
Left primary bronchus
Intercostal v.
Intercostal a.
Intercostal n.
Pulmonary v.
Ninth rib
Diaphragm
Costodiaphragmatic recess
Spleen
Left kidney

The plane of section passes to the left side of the median plane and
passes through the costal cartilages at their junction with the sternum.

Sagittal Section

THORAX.   Plate 3-1

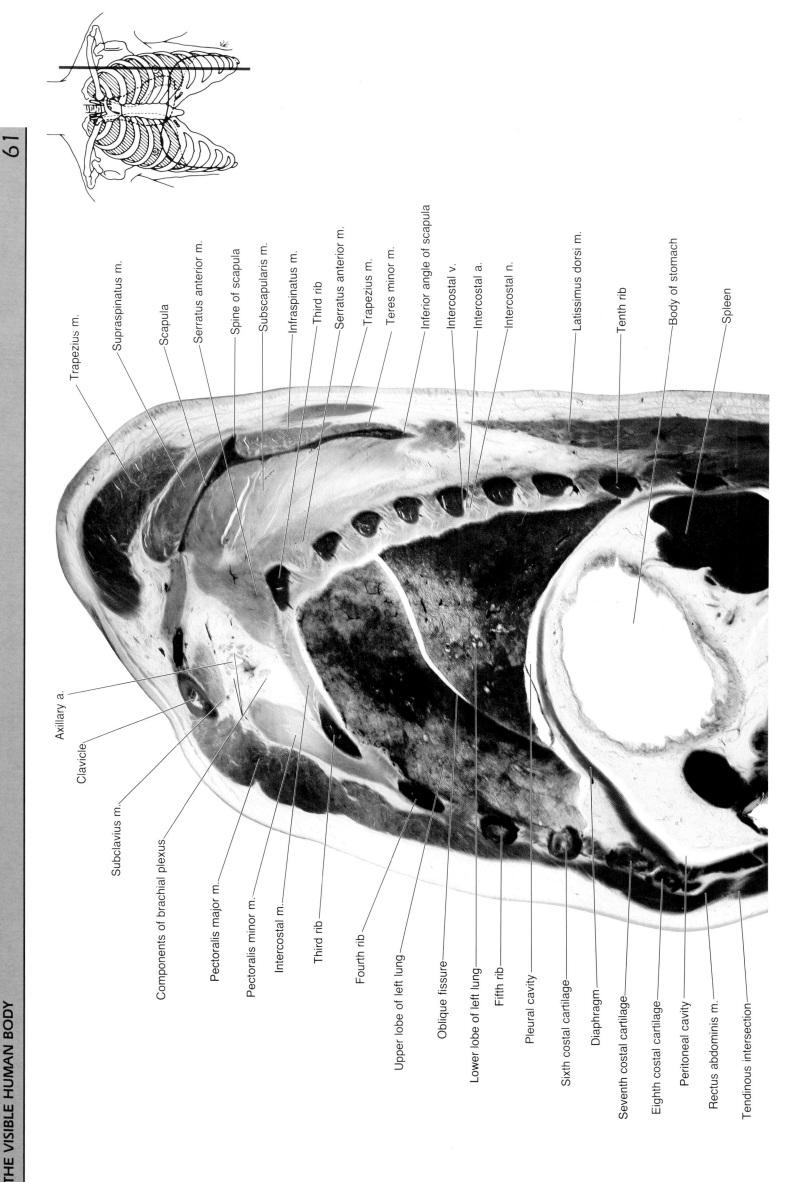

Trapezius m.

Supraspinatus m.

Scapula

Serratus anterior m.

Spine of scapula

Subscapularis m.

Infraspinatus m.

Third rib

Serratus anterior m.

Trapezius m.

Teres minor m.

Inferior angle of scapula

Intercostal v.

Intercostal a.

Intercostal n.

Latissimus dorsi m.

Tenth rib

Body of stomach

Spleen

Axillary a.

Clavicle

Subclavius m.

Components of brachial plexus

Pectoralis major m.

Pectoralis minor m.

Intercostal m.

Third rib

Fourth rib

Upper lobe of left lung

Oblique fissure

Lower lobe of left lung

Fifth rib

Pleural cavity

Sixth costal cartilage

Diaphragm

Seventh costal cartilage

Eighth costal cartilage

Peritoneal cavity

Rectus abdominis m.

Tendinous intersection

The plane of section passes approximately 10 cm to the left of the median plane and passes through the axilla.

THORAX.   Plate 3-2

Sagittal Section

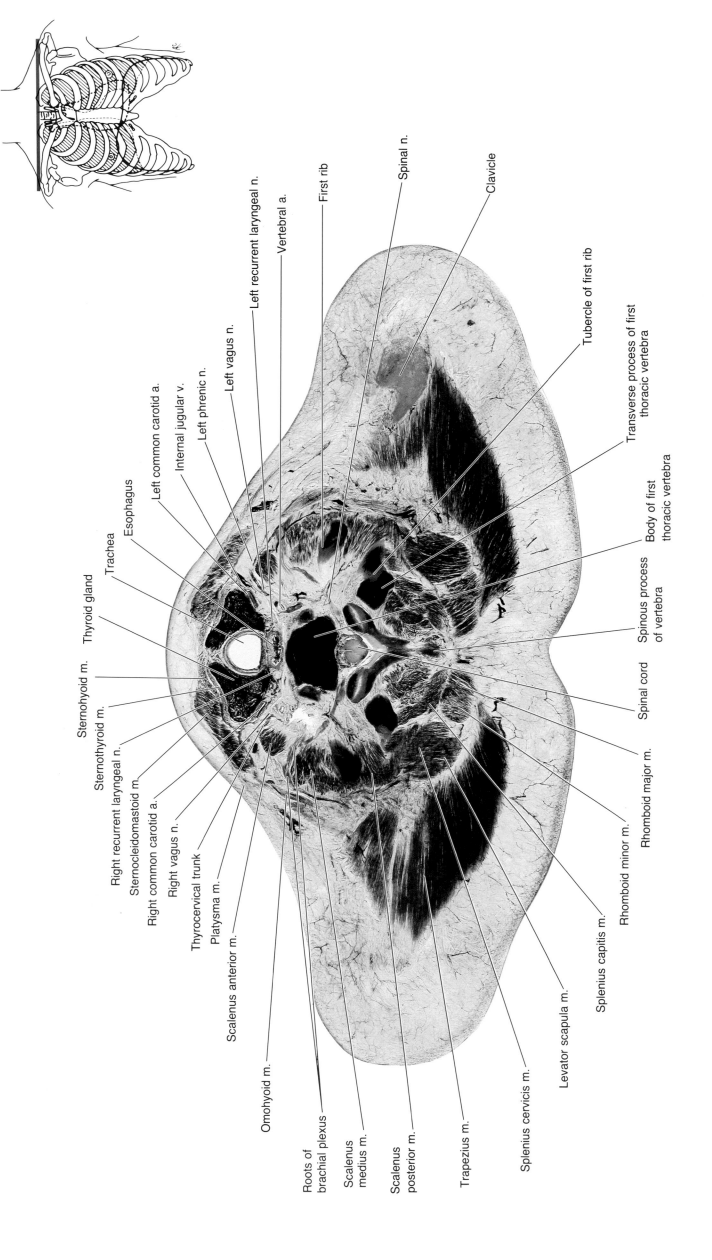

Left recurrent laryngeal n.

Vertebral a.

Spinal n.

First rib

Clavicle

Tubercle of first rib

Transverse process of first thoracic vertebra

Body of first thoracic vertebra

Spinous process of vertebra

Spinal cord

Rhomboid major m.

Rhomboid minor m.

Splenius capitis m.

Levator scapula m.

Splenius cervicis m.

Trapezius m.

Scalenus posterior m.

Scalenus medius m.

Roots of brachial plexus

Omohyoid m.

Scalenus anterior m.

Platysma m.

Thyrocervical trunk

Right vagus n.

Right common carotid a.

Sternocleidomastoid m.

Right recurrent laryngeal n.

Sternothyroid m.

Sternohyoid m.

Thyroid gland

Trachea

Esophagus

Left common carotid a.

Internal jugular v.

Left phrenic n.

Left vagus n.

THORAX. Plate 3-3

The plane of section passes through the root of the neck at the level of the first thoracic vertebra and the head of the first rib.

Transverse Section

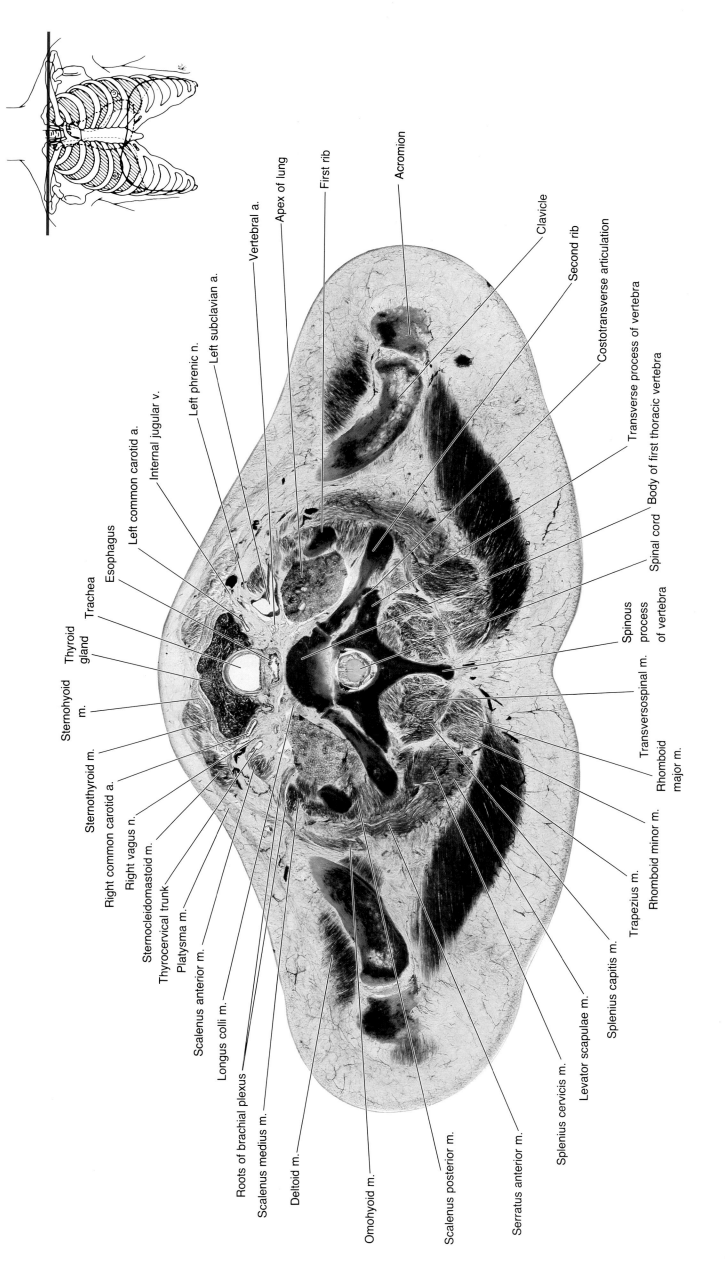

Vertebral a.

Apex of lung

First rib

Acromion

Clavicle

Second rib

Costotransverse articulation

Transverse process of vertebra

Body of first thoracic vertebra

Spinal cord

Spinous process of vertebra

Transversospinal m.

Rhomboid major m.

Rhomboid minor m.

Trapezius m.

Splenius capitis m.

Levator scapulae m.

Splenius cervicis m.

Scalenus posterior m.

Serratus anterior m.

Left phrenic n.

Left subclavian a.

Internal jugular v.

Left common carotid a.

Esophagus

Trachea

Thyroid gland

Sternohyoid m.

Sternothyroid m.

Right common carotid a.

Right vagus n.

Thyrocervical trunk

Sternocleidomastoid m.

Platysma m.

Scalenus anterior m.

Longus colli m.

Roots of brachial plexus

Scalenus medius m.

Deltoid m.

Omohyoid m.

THORAX. Plate 3-4

Transverse Section

The plane of section passes through the apex of the lungs at the level of the lower edge of the first thoracic vertebra and the head of the second rib.

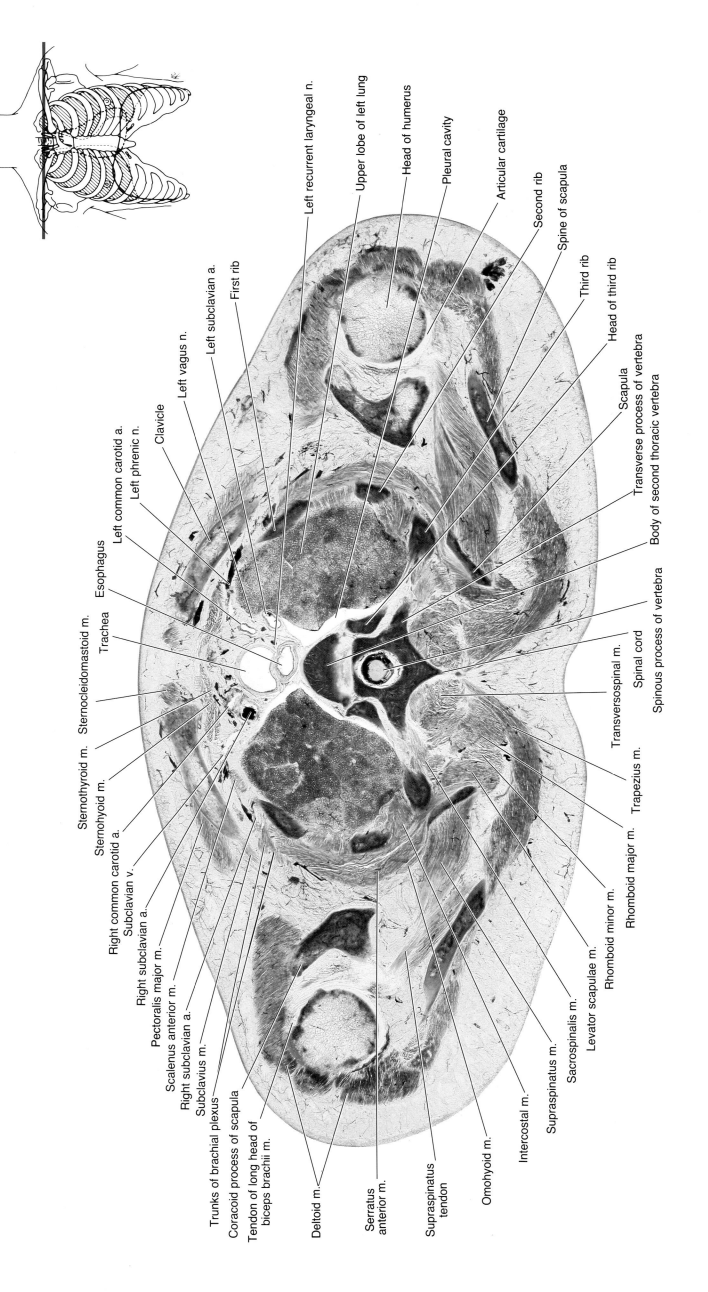

Left recurrent laryngeal n.

Upper lobe of left lung

Head of humerus

Pleural cavity

Articular cartilage

Second rib

Spine of scapula

Third rib

Head of third rib

Scapula

Transverse process of vertebra

Body of second thoracic vertebra

Spinous process of vertebra

Spinal cord

Transversospinal m.

Trapezius m.

Rhomboid minor m.

Rhomboid major m.

Levator scapulae m.

Sacrospinalis m.

Supraspinatus m.

Intercostal m.

Omohyoid m.

Supraspinatus tendon

Serratus anterior m.

Deltoid m.

Tendon of long head of biceps brachii m.

Coracoid process of scapula

Trunks of brachial plexus

Subclavius m.

Right subclavian a.

Scalenus anterior m.

Pectoralis major m.

Right subclavian a.

Subclavian v.

Right common carotid a.

Sternothyroid m.

Sternohyoid m.

Sternocleidomastoid m.

Trachea

Esophagus

Left common carotid a.

Left phrenic n.

Clavicle

Left vagus n.

Left subclavian a.

First rib

THORAX. Plate 3-5

Tranverse Section

The plane of section passes through the superior mediastinum at the level of the second thoracic vertebra and above the branching of the brachiocephalic artery.

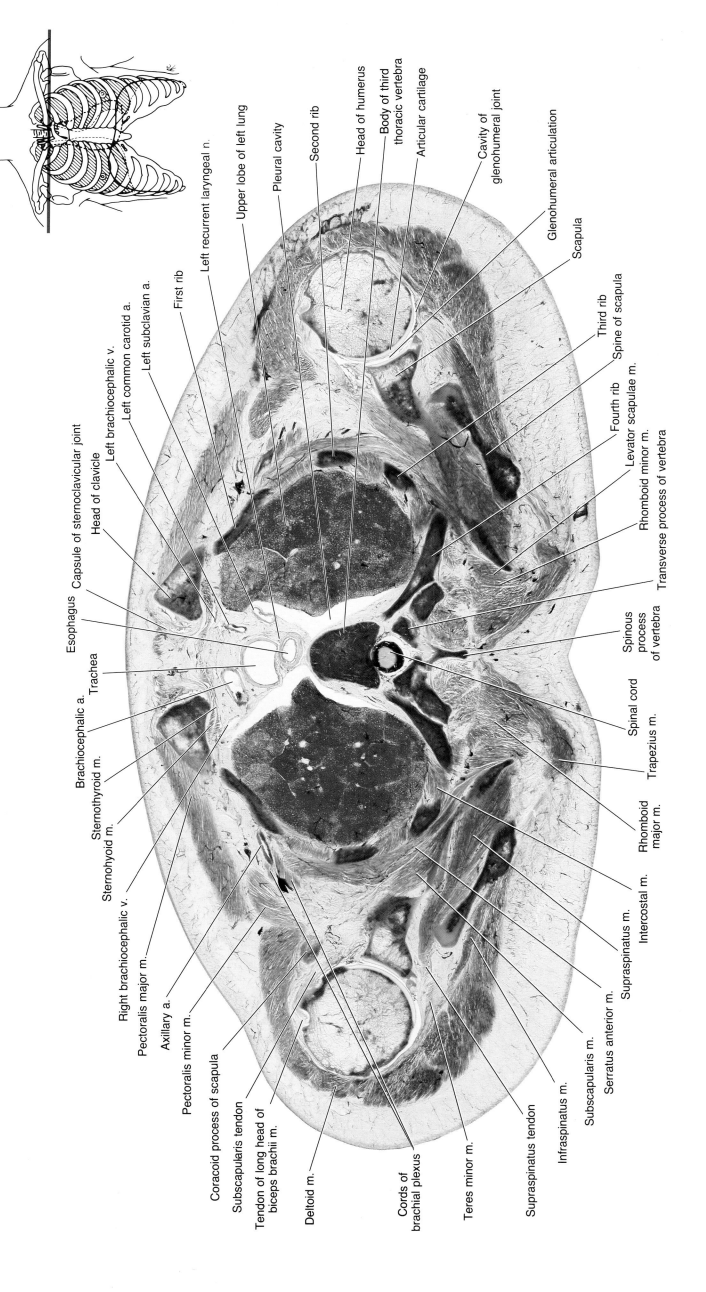

Left recurrent laryngeal n.
Upper lobe of left lung
Pleural cavity
Second rib
Head of humerus
Body of third thoracic vertebra
Articular cartilage
Cavity of glenohumeral joint
Glenohumeral articulation
Scapula

First rib
Left subclavian a.
Left common carotid a.
Left brachiocephalic v.
Head of clavicle
Capsule of sternoclavicular joint
Esophagus

Third rib
Spine of scapula
Fourth rib
Levator scapulae m.
Rhomboid minor m.
Transverse process of vertebra

Brachiocephalic a.
Trachea
Sternothyroid m.
Sternohyoid m.
Right brachiocephalic v.
Pectoralis major m.
Axillary a.
Pectoralis minor m.

Spinous process of vertebra
Spinal cord
Trapezius m.

Coracoid process of scapula
Subscapularis tendon
Tendon of long head of biceps brachii m.
Deltoid m.
Cords of brachial plexus
Teres minor m.
Supraspinatus tendon
Infraspinatus m.
Subscapularis m.
Serratus anterior m.
Supraspinatus m.
Intercostal m.
Rhomboid major m.

THORAX.
Plate 3-6

Transverse Section

The plane of section passes through the superior mediastinum at the level of the third thoracic vertebra and the major vessels arising from the aortic arch.

Left brachiocephalic v.

Right brachiocephalic v.

Pectoralis major m.

Pectoralis minor m.

Trachea

Esophagus

Manubrium

Brachiocephalic a.

Left common carotid a.

Left subclavian a.

Body of fourth thoracic vertebra

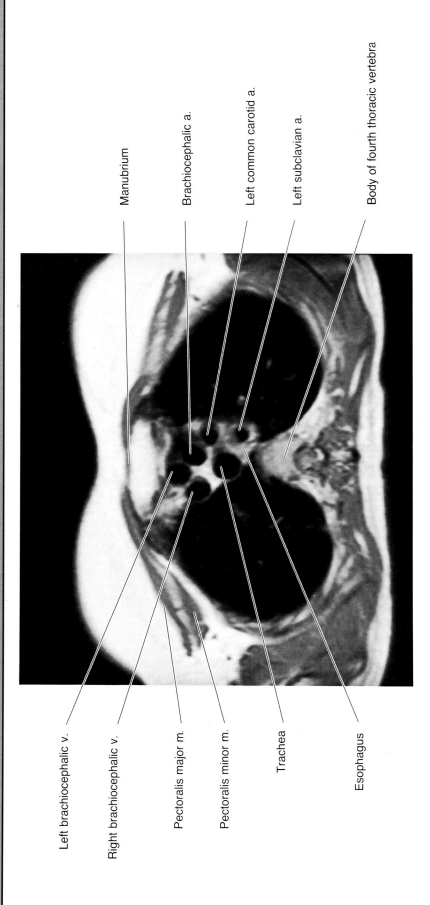

The sections shown in Plate 3-7 and the accompanying MRI (Plate 3-7 MRI) pass in a transverse plane through the superior mediastinum at the level of the fourth thoracic vertebra. The plane in Plate 3-7 MRI passes through the superior mediastinum immediately above the aortic arch; the plane of section in Plate 3-7 is slightly below this level and includes the posterior portion of the aortic arch. The three major arteries arising from the aortic arch, namely the brachiocephalic, left common carotid, and left subclavian arteries, can be identified in Plate 3-7 MRI. The left subclavian artery is not included in the section in Plate 3-7 because the plane of the section passes through the posterior portion of the aortic arch. The position of the three arteries, as they arise from the aortic arch (see Plate 3-7 MRI), indicates the course of the aortic arch as it arises from the ascending aorta on the right side of the trachea and passes in a diagonal plane from anterior to posterior. The aortic arch passes anterior and to the left of the trachea. At the level of the sternal angle, the arch becomes continuous with the descending aorta which lies anterior and on the left side of the vertebral body. In both plates the right and left brachiocephalic veins can be identified anterior to the arteries arising from the aortic arch.

Four structures, the trachea, esophagus, left recurrent laryngeal nerve, and thoracic duct, pass in parallel through the mediastinum. The U-shaped trachea can be seen as it lies posterior to the aortic arch and its branches. The esophagus lies adjacent to the flattened posterior surface of the trachea and the left recurrent laryngeal nerve runs in the angle between these two structures. These three structures are identified in Plate 3-7. The thin-walled thoracic duct, which passes through the superior mediastinum on the left side of the esophagus, cannot be identified in the section.

The plane of section also passes through the axilla. In Plate 3-7, the axillary artery and associated cords of the brachial plexus are identified. The anterior wall of the axilla is formed by the pectoralis major and minor muscles. The serratus anterior muscle, ribs, and intercostal muscles form the medial wall. The posterior wall is formed by the subscapularis, teres major, and latissimus dorsi muscles. Lymph nodes can be seen embedded in the fat within the axilla. The long and short heads of the biceps muscle and the coracobrachialis muscle can also be identified in the axilla.

Plate 3-7 MRI
Transverse Section

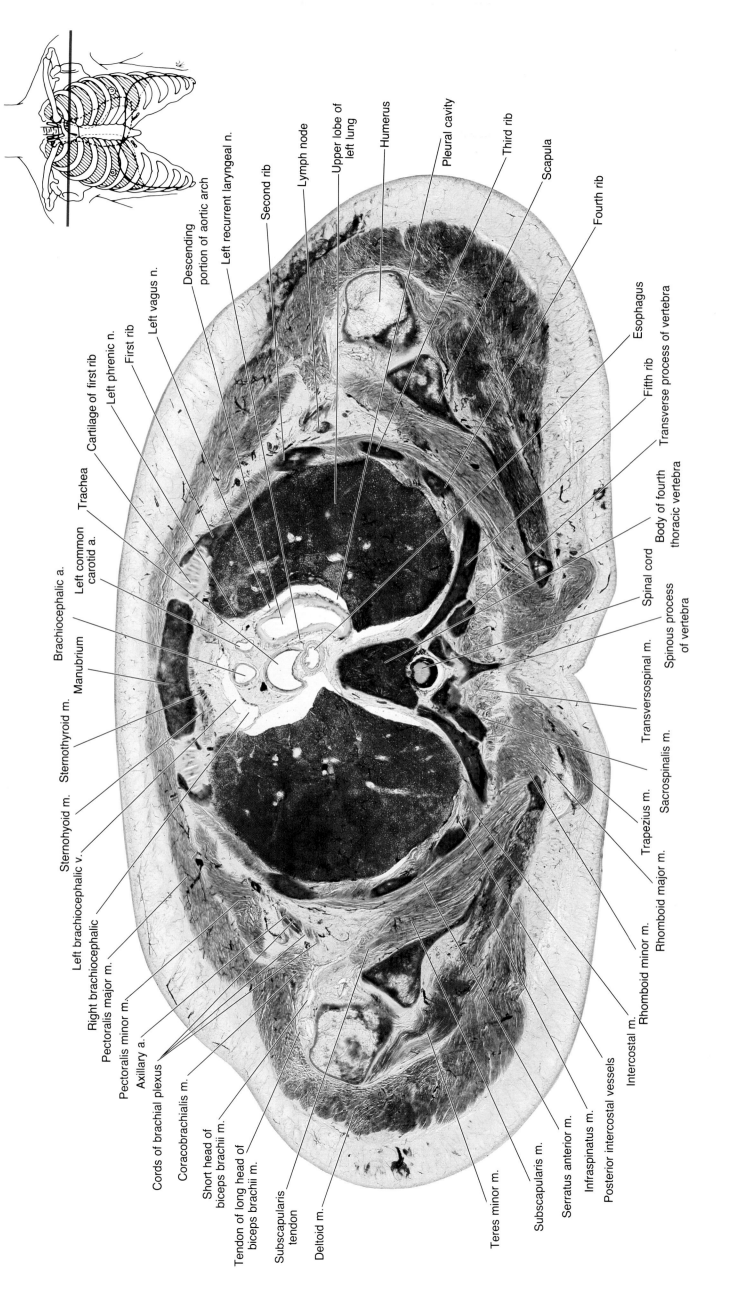

Humerus

Pleural cavity

Third rib

Scapula

Fourth rib

Upper lobe of left lung

Lymph node

Second rib

Left recurrent laryngeal n.

Descending portion of aortic arch

Left vagus n.

First rib

Left phrenic n.

Cartilage of first rib

Trachea

Brachiocephalic a.

Left common carotid a.

Manubrium

Sternothyroid m.

Sternohyoid m.

Left brachiocephalic v.

Right brachiocephalic

Pectoralis major m.

Pectoralis minor m.

Axillary a.

Cords of brachial plexus

Coracobrachialis m.

Short head of biceps brachii m.

Tendon of long head of biceps brachii m.

Subscapularis tendon

Deltoid m.

Teres minor m.

Subscapularis m.

Serratus anterior m.

Infraspinatus m.

Posterior intercostal vessels

Intercostal m.

Rhomboid minor m.

Rhomboid major m.

Trapezius m.

Sacrospinalis m.

Transversospinal m.

Spinous process of vertebra

Spinal cord

Body of fourth thoracic vertebra

Transverse process of vertebra

Fifth rib

Esophagus

The plane of section passes through the superior mediastinum at the level of the fourth thoracic vertebra and the superior border of the aortic arch.

Transverse Section

THORAX. Plate 3-7

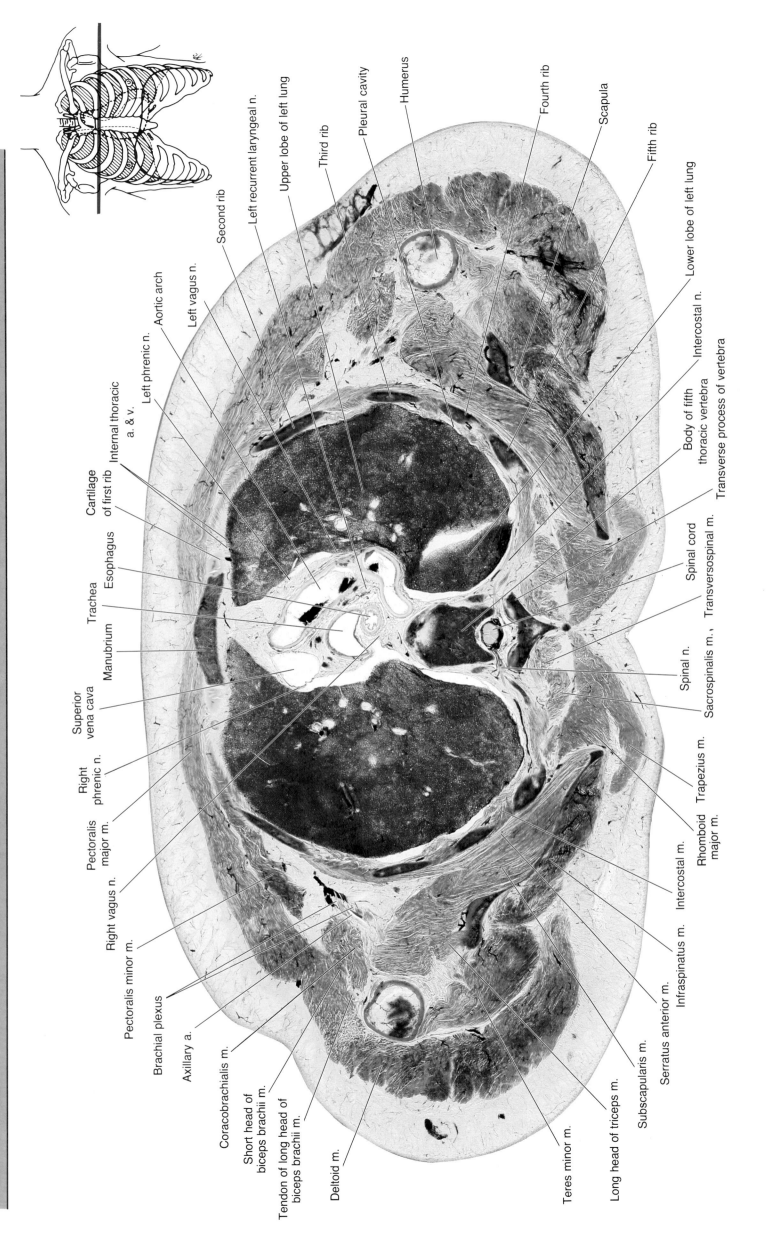

Second rib

Left recurrent laryngeal n.

Upper lobe of left lung

Third rib

Pleural cavity

Humerus

Fourth rib

Scapula

Fifth rib

Lower lobe of left lung

Intercostal n.

Transverse process of vertebra

Body of fifth thoracic vertebra

Left vagus n.

Aortic arch

Left phrenic n.

Internal thoracic a. & v.

Cartilage of first rib

Esophagus

Trachea

Manubrium

Superior vena cava

Right phrenic n.

Right vagus n.

Pectoralis minor m.

Brachial plexus

Axillary a.

Coracobrachialis m.

Short head of biceps brachii m.

Tendon of long head of biceps brachii m.

Deltoid m.

Spinal cord

Transversospinal m.

Spinal n.

Sacrospinalis m. ,

Trapezius m.

Rhomboid major m.

Intercostal m.

Infraspinatus m.

Serratus anterior m.

Subscapularis m.

Long head of triceps m.

Teres minor m.

Pectoralis major m.

THORAX.   Plate 3-8

Transverse Section

The plane of section passes through the superior mediastinum at the level of the fifth thoracic vertebra and the aortic arch.

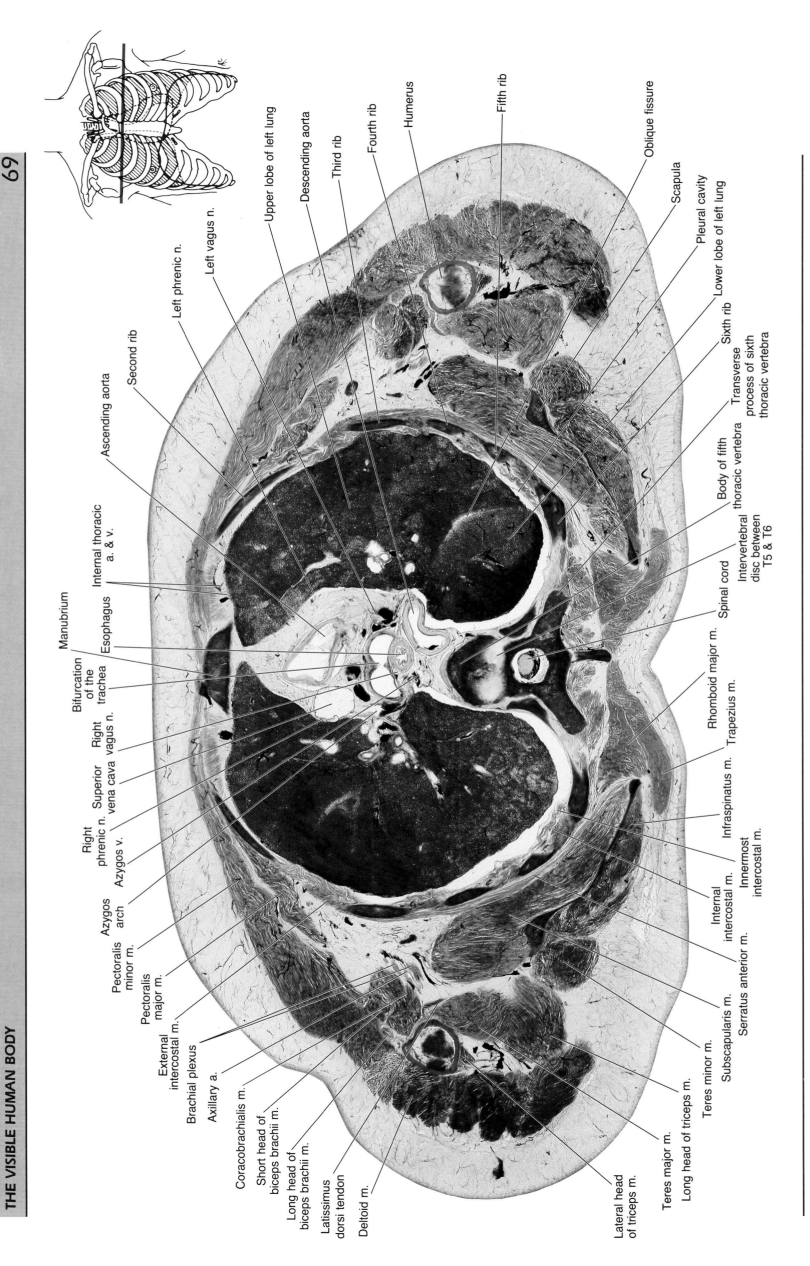

Upper lobe of left lung
Descending aorta
Third rib
Fourth rib
Humerus
Fifth rib
Oblique fissure
Scapula
Pleural cavity
Lower lobe of left lung
Sixth rib
Transverse process of sixth thoracic vertebra
Body of fifth thoracic vertebra
Intervertebral disc between T5 & T6
Spinal cord
Rhomboid major m.
Trapezius m.
Infraspinatus m.
Innermost intercostal m.
Internal intercostal m.
Subscapularis m.
Serratus anterior m.
Teres minor m.
Long head of triceps m.
Teres major m.
Lateral head of triceps m.
Deltoid m.
Latissimus dorsi tendon
Long head of biceps brachii m.
Short head of biceps brachii m.
Coracobrachialis m.
Axillary a.
Brachial plexus
External intercostal m.
Pectoralis major m.
Pectoralis minor m.
Azygos arch
Azygos v.
Superior vena cava
Right phrenic n.
Right vagus n.
Bifurcation of the trachea
Esophagus
Manubrium
Internal thoracic a. & v.
Ascending aorta
Second rib
Left vagus n.
Left phrenic n.

THORAX.   Plate 3-9

Transverse Section

The plane of section passes through the inferior mediastinum at the level of the intervertebral disc between T5 and T6 and the bifurcation of the trachea.

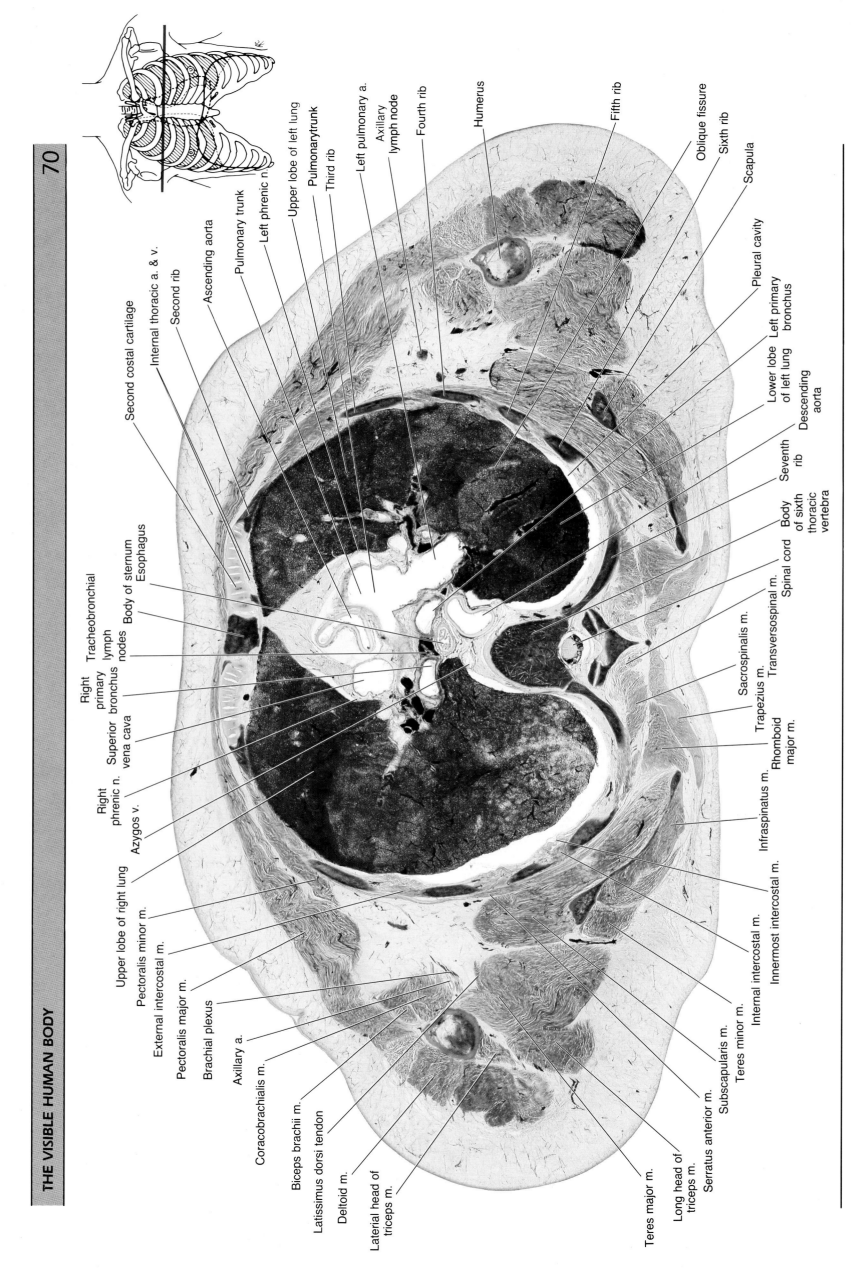

Second costal cartilage
Internal thoracic a. & v.
Second rib
Ascending aorta
Pulmonary trunk
Left phrenic n.
Upper lobe of left lung
Pulmonarytrunk
Third rib
Left pulmonary a.
Axillary lymph node
Fourth rib
Humerus
Fifth rib
Oblique fissure
Sixth rib
Scapula
Pleural cavity
Left primary bronchus
Lower lobe of left lung
Descending aorta
Seventh rib
Body of sixth thoracic vertebra
Spinal cord
Transversospinal m.
Sacrospinalis m.
Trapezius m.
Rhomboid major m.
Infraspinatus m.
Internal intercostal m.
Innermost intercostal m.
Teres minor m.
Subscapularis m.
Serratus anterior m.
Long head of triceps m.
Teres major m.

Esophagus
Body of sternum
Tracheobronchial lymph nodes
Right primary bronchus
Right phrenic n.
Superior vena cava
Azygos v.
Upper lobe of right lung
Pectoralis minor m.
External intercostal m.
Pectoralis major m.
Deltoid m.
Brachial plexus
Axillary a.
Coracobrachialis m.
Biceps brachii m.
Latissimus dorsi tendon
Lateral head of triceps m.

THORAX.   Plate 3-10   Transverse Section

The plane of section passes through the inferior mediastinum at the level of the sixth thoracic vertebra, pulmonary trunk, and left pulmonary artery.

Internal thoracic a. & v.

Upper lobe of left lung

Pulmonary trunk

Third rib

Left phrenic n.

Pulmonary v.

Left secondary bronchi

Fourth rib

Descending aorta

Fifth rib

Humerus

Pleural cavity

Sixth rib

Lower lobe of left lung

Scapula

Seventh rib

Seventh thoracic vertebra

Spinal cord

Spinous process of sixth thoracic vertebra

Transversospinal m.

Sacrospinalis m.

Rhomboid major m.

Trapezius m.

Internal intercostal m.

Innermost intercostal m.

Teres minor m.

Subscapularis m.

Serratus anterior m.

Teres major m.

Latissimus dorsi m.

Ulnar n.

Long head of triceps m.

Radial n.

Lateral head of triceps m.

Axillary a.

Median n.

Biceps brachii m.

Coracobrachialis m.

Deltoid m.

Pectoralis major m.

Oblique fissure

External intercostal m.

Pectoralis minor m.

Pectoralis major m.

Right primary bronchus

Azygos v.

Right phrenic n.

Right pulmonary a.

Upper lobe of right lung

Superior vena cava

Body of sternum

Esophagus

Ascending aorta

THORAX.   Plate 3-11

Transverse Section

The plane of section passes through the inferior mediastinum at the level of the seventh thoracic vertebra, pulmonary trunk, and right plumonary artery.

Body of sternum

Pulmonary trunk

Left atrium

Esophagus

Descending aorta

Ascending aorta

Superior vena cava

Right pulmonary v.

Azygos v.

Body of seventh thoracic vertebra

The sections shown in Plate 3-12 and the accompanying MRI (Plate 3-12 MRI) pass in a transverse plane through the inferior mediastinum at the level of the seventh thoracic vertebra. The plane of the section shown in Plate 3-12 MRI passes through the inferior mediastinum slightly above the plane of the section in Plate 3-12. The left atrium forms the base of the heart and is identified in both plates. In the MRI the right superior pulmonary vein is included in the section as it joins the left atrium. In Plate 3-12 the right inferior and left superior pulmonary veins are included in the plane of section as it passes through the left atrium. In both plates the superior vena cava can be seen. In the MRI the section includes the proximal portion of the ascending aorta and the base of the pulmonary trunk. However, in Plate 3-12 the plane of section is slightly lower and passes through the ascending aorta immediately above the aortic valve, through the base of the pulmonary trunk at the level of the pulmonic valve, such that portions of the cusps of the valve are included, and also through the right auricle.

In the posterior mediastinum, the esophagus lies posterior to the left atrium adjacent to the posterior wall of the pericardial sac. The descending aorta lies posterior and to the left of the esophagus. The azygos vein can also be seen as it lies immediately anterior to the vertebral body.

Enlarged lymph nodes can be seen in the anterior mediastinum and in the floor of the axilla. This is a result of a malignant melanoma which in this individual metastasized to widely dispersed locations including the liver, lymph nodes of the axilla, inguinal region, and thoracic cavity and also involved bones throughout the body.

Plate 3-12 MRI
Transverse Section

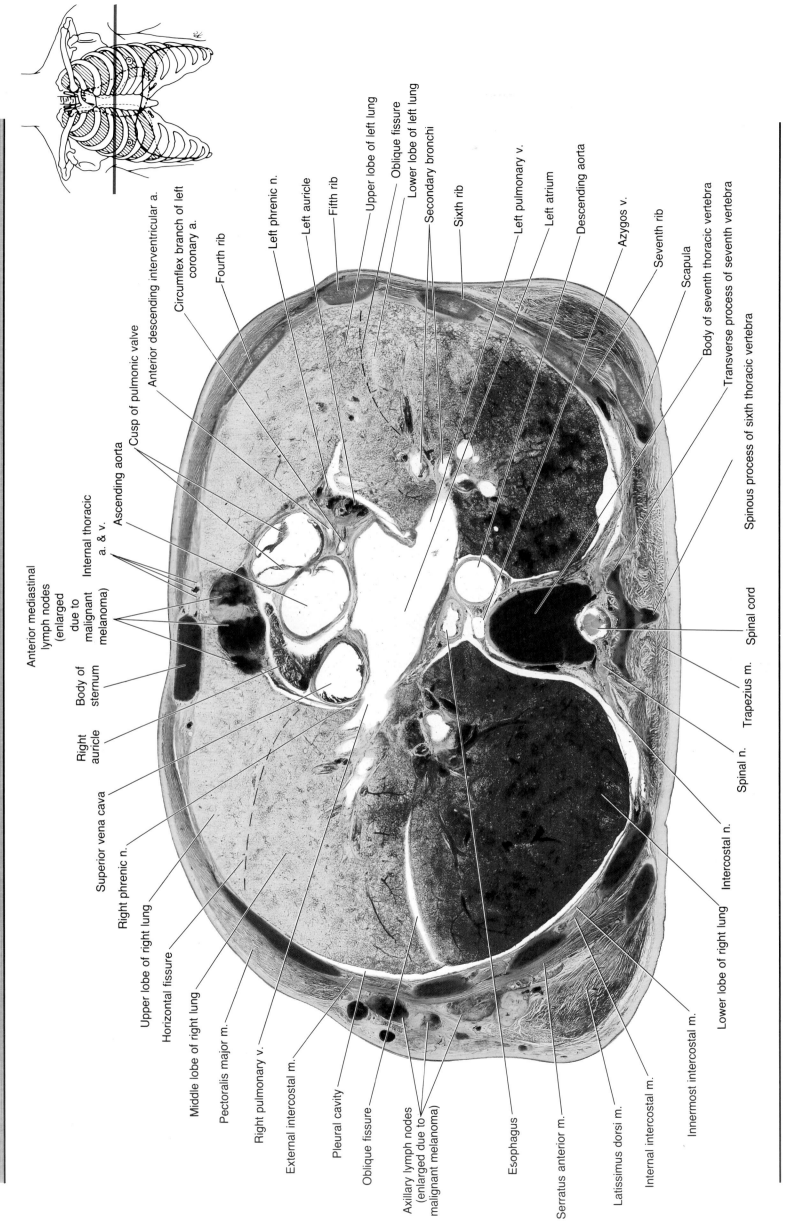

Anterior mediastinal lymph nodes (enlarged due to malignant melanoma)

Internal thoracic a. & v.

Ascending aorta

Cusp of pulmonic valve

Anterior descending interventricular a.

Circumflex branch of left coronary a.

Fourth rib

Left phrenic n.

Left auricle

Fifth rib

Upper lobe of left lung

Oblique fissure

Lower lobe of left lung

Secondary bronchi

Sixth rib

Left pulmonary v.

Left atrium

Descending aorta

Azygos v.

Seventh rib

Scapula

Body of seventh thoracic vertebra

Transverse process of seventh vertebra

Spinous process of sixth thoracic vertebra

Spinal cord

Trapezius m.

Spinal n.

Intercostal n.

Esophagus

Serratus anterior m.

Latissimus dorsi m.

Internal intercostal m.

Innermost intercostal m.

Lower lobe of right lung

Axillary lymph nodes (enlarged due to malignant melanoma)

Oblique fissure

Pleural cavity

External intercostal m.

Right pulmonary v.

Pectoralis major m.

Middle lobe of right lung

Horizontal fissure

Upper lobe of right lung

Right phrenic n.

Superior vena cava

Right auricle

Body of sternum

The plane of section passes through the inferior mediastinum at the level of the seventh thoracic vertebra and the pulmonic valve.

Transverse Section

THORAX.   Plate 3-12

Body of sternum

Right ventricle

Esophagus

Left pulmonary v.

Segmental bronchi

Descending aorta

Body of seventh thoracic vertebra

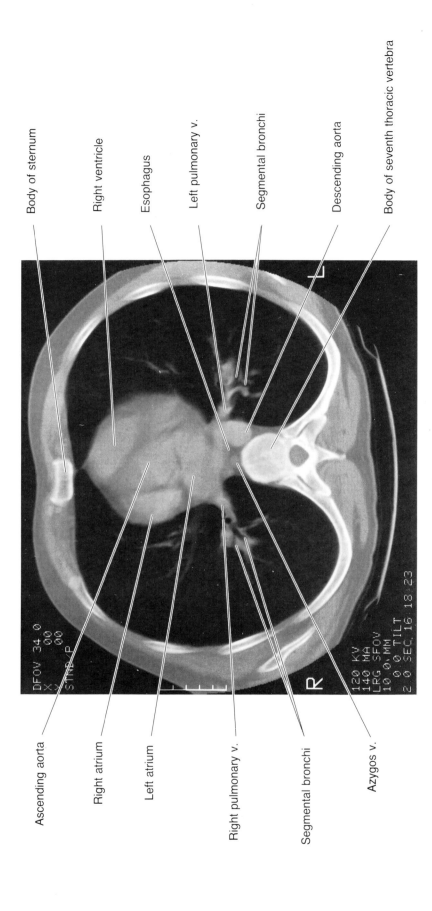

Ascending aorta

Right atrium

Left atrium

Right pulmonary v.

Segmental bronchi

Azygos v.

The sections shown in Plate 3-13 and the accompanying CT (Plate 3-13 CT) pass in a transverse plane through the inferior mediastinum at the level of the seventh thoracic vertebra. The plane in Plate 3-13 CT passes through the inferior mediastinum slightly above the plane of the section in plate 3-13. The left atrium forms the base of the heart. In the plane shown in the CT, the pulmonary veins can be identified as they join the left atrium. In Plate 3-13, the right pulmonary vein is identified, however the plane of section passes below the level of the left pulmonary vein. The right atrium is identified in both sections as is the right ventricle. The portion of the right ventricle included in Plate 3-13 is the conus arteriosus. In the CT, the plane of section passes through the ascending aorta. However, in Plate 3-13 the section is slightly below this level and passes through the aortic valve. Therefore, the cusps of the aortic valve can be seen. To the left of the aortic valve, a portion of the left ventricular wall is included in the section. In Plate 3-13, it is also possible to identify the fossa ovalis, coronary sinus, right coronary artery, and the circumflex and anterior descending branches of the left coronary artery.

In the posterior mediastinum, the esophagus lies adjacent to the posterior wall of the pericardium. In Plate 3-13 the esophagus can be seen, as it lies in the median sagittal plane, posterior to the left atrium. The descending aorta lies posterior and to the left of the esophagus. The azygos and hemiazygos veins can also be seen as they lie immediately anterior to the verbral body. The esophagus, azygos vein, and descending aorta can also be identified in Plate 3-13 CT.

Enlarged lymph nodes can be seen in the anterior mediastinum. This is a result of malignant melanoma, which in this individual was widely dispersed in lymph nodes of the axilla, inguinal region, and thoracic cavity and also involved the liver and bones throughout the body.

Plate 3-13 CT
Transverse Section

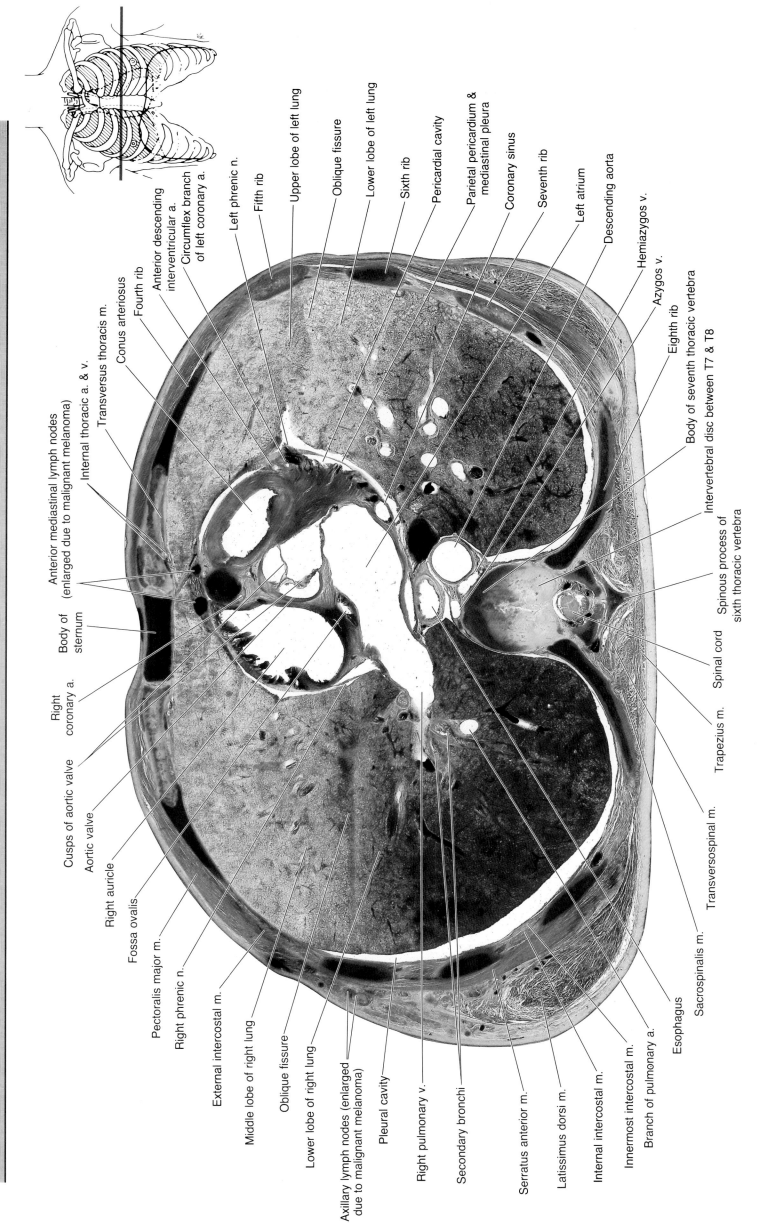

Upper lobe of left lung
Oblique fissure
Lower lobe of left lung
Sixth rib
Pericardial cavity
Parietal pericardium & mediastinal pleura
Coronary sinus
Seventh rib
Left atrium
Descending aorta
Hemiazygos v.
Azygos v.
Eighth rib
Body of seventh thoracic vertebra
Intervertebral disc between T7 & T8
Spinal cord
Spinous process of sixth thoracic vertebra
Trapezius m.
Transversospinal m.
Sacrospinalis m.
Esophagus
Branch of pulmonary a.
Innermost intercostal m.
Internal intercostal m.
Latissimus dorsi m.
Serratus anterior m.
Secondary bronchi
Right pulmonary v.
Pleural cavity
Lower lobe of right lung
Oblique fissure
Middle lobe of right lung
External intercostal m.
Right phrenic n.
Pectoralis major m.
Fossa ovalis
Right auricle
Aortic valve
Cusps of aortic valve
Right coronary a.
Body of sternum
Axillary lymph nodes (enlarged due to malignant melanoma)
Anterior mediastinal lymph nodes (enlarged due to malignant melanoma)
Internal thoracic a. & v.
Transversus thoracis m.
Conus arteriosus
Fourth rib
Anterior descending interventricular a.
Circumflex branch of left coronary a.
Left phrenic n.
Fifth rib

THORAX.   Plate 3-13

Transverse Section

The plane of section passes through the inferior mediastinum at the level of the intervertebral disc between T7 and T8 and the aortic valve.

Interventricular septum

Left ventricle

Cusps of mitral valve

Esophagus

Descending aorta

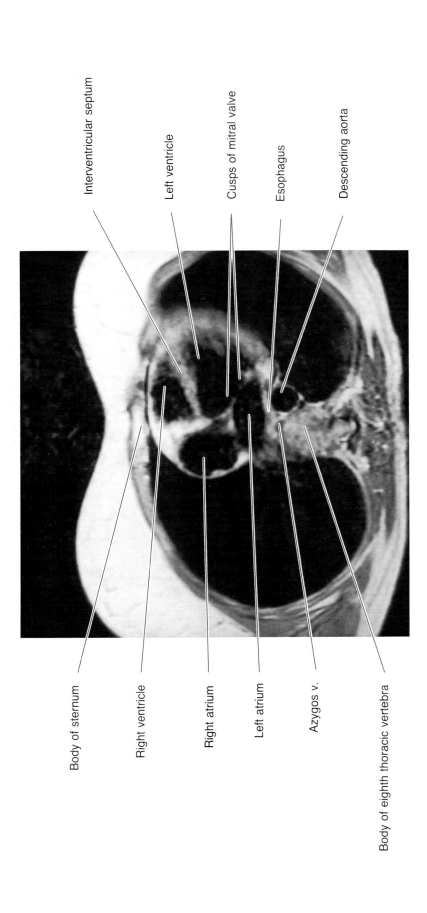

Body of sternum

Right ventricle

Right atrium

Left atrium

Azygos v.

Body of eighth thoracic vertebra

The sections shown in Plate 3-14 and the accompanying MRI (Plate 3-14 MRI) pass in a transverse plane through the inferior mediastinum at the level of the eight thoracic vertebra. The plane in Plate 3-14 MRI passes through the inferior mediastinum slightly above the plane of the section in plate 3-14. All four chambers of the heart can be identified in both plates. In Plate 3-14 the section passes through both of the atrioventricular orifices and, therefore, cusps of tricuspid and mitral (or bicuspid) valves can be seen. In the MRI the plane of section is slightly above the level of the tricuspid valve; however, the cusps of the mitral valve are clearly visible. In both sections the right and left atria and the interventricular and interatrial septa are identified. In Plate 3-14, it is also possible to identify the coronary sinus, right coronary artery, and the circumflex and anterior descending branches of the left coronary arteries.

In both plates the esophagus, descending aorta, and azygos vein can be identified in the posterior mediastinum. In Plate 3-14 the esophagus can be seen, as it lies in the median sagittal plane, posterior to the left atrium with the descending aorta lying posterior and to the left side. The thoracic duct and azygos and hemiazygos veins can also be seen as they lie anterior to the vertebral body. In Plate 3-14 enlarged lymph nodes can be seen in the anterior mediastinum due to the presence of metastatic malignant melanoma (see Plate 3-13 CT).

Plate 3-14 MRI
Transverse Section

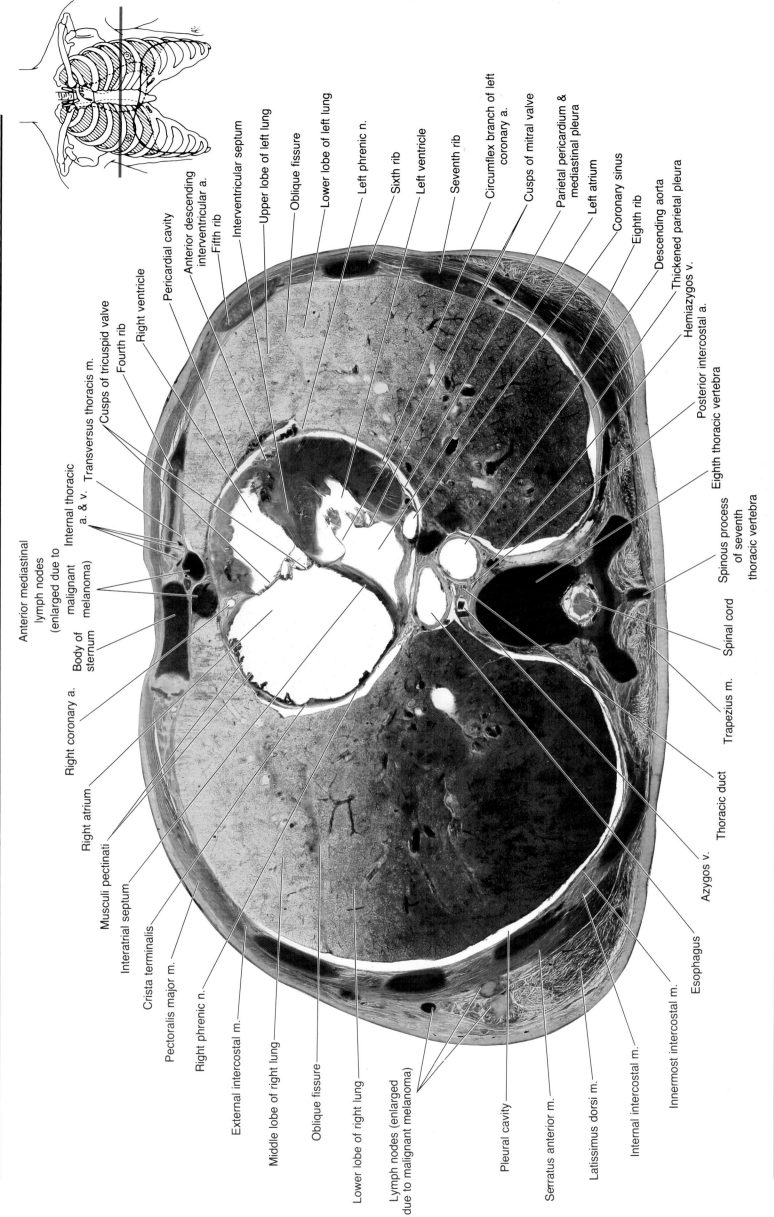

Anterior mediastinal
lymph nodes
(enlarged due to
malignant melanoma)

Internal thoracic
a. & v.

Body of
sternum

Transversus thoracis m.

Cusps of tricuspid valve

Fourth rib

Right ventricle

Pericardial cavity

Anterior descending
interventricular a.

Fifth rib

Interventricular septum

Upper lobe of left lung

Oblique fissure

Lower lobe of left lung

Left phrenic n.

Sixth rib

Left ventricle

Seventh rib

Circumflex branch of left
coronary a.

Cusps of mitral valve

Parietal pericardium &
mediastinal pleura

Left atrium

Coronary sinus

Eighth rib

Descending aorta

Thickened parietal pleura

Hemiazygos v.

Posterior intercostal a.

Eighth thoracic vertebra

Spinous process
of seventh
thoracic vertebra

Spinal cord

Trapezius m.

Thoracic duct

Azygos v.

Esophagus

Innermost intercostal m.

Internal intercostal m.

Latissimus dorsi m.

Serratus anterior m.

Pleural cavity

Lymph nodes (enlarged
due to malignant melanoma)

Oblique fissure

Lower lobe of right lung

Middle lobe of right lung

External intercostal m.

Pectoralis major m.

Right phrenic n.

Crista terminalis

Interatrial septum

Musculi pectinati

Right atrium

Right coronary a.

THORAX.   Plate 3-14

The plane of section passes through the inferior mediastinum at the level of the
eighth thoracic vertebra and the mitral and tricuspid valves of the heart.

Transverse Section

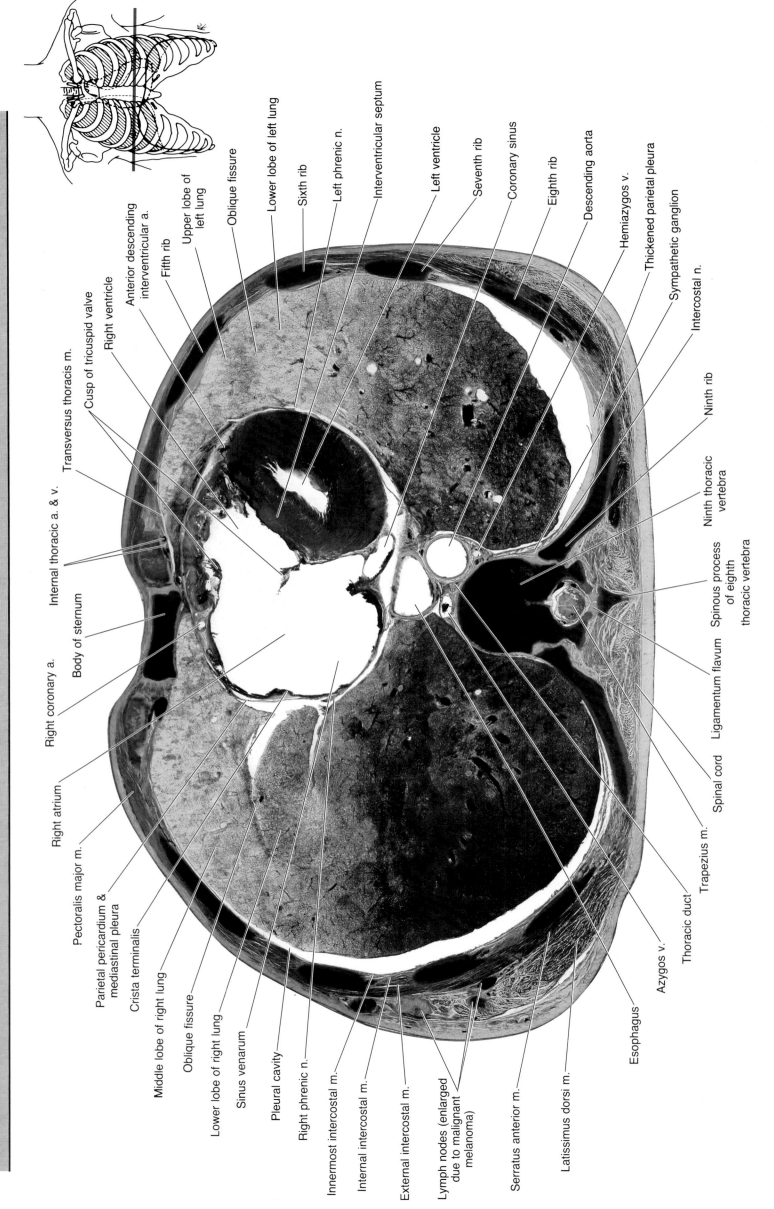

Upper lobe of left lung

Oblique fissure

Lower lobe of left lung

Sixth rib

Left phrenic n.

Interventricular septum

Left ventricle

Seventh rib

Coronary sinus

Eighth rib

Descending aorta

Hemiazygos v.

Thickened parietal pleura

Sympathetic ganglion

Intercostal n.

Ninth rib

Ninth thoracic vertebra

Spinous process of eighth thoracic vertebra

Cusp of tricuspid valve

Right ventricle

Anterior descending interventricular a.

Fifth rib

Transversus thoracis m.

Internal thoracic a. & v.

Body of sternum

Right coronary a.

Pectoralis major m.

Parietal pericardium & mediastinal pleura

Crista terminalis

Right atrium

Middle lobe of right lung

Oblique fissure

Lower lobe of right lung

Sinus venarum

Pleural cavity

Right phrenic n.

Innermost intercostal m.

Internal intercostal m.

External intercostal m.

Lymph nodes (enlarged due to malignant melanoma)

Serratus anterior m.

Latissimus dorsi m.

Esophagus

Azygos v.

Thoracic duct

Trapezius m.

Spinal cord

Ligamentum flavum

THORAX.   Plate 3-15

Transverse Section

The plane of section passes through the inferior mediastinum at the level of the upper border of the ninth thoracic vertebra and the opening of the coronary sinus.

Valve of the coronary sinus
Pectoralis major m.
Right atrium

Parietal pericardium & mediastinal pleura
Valve of the inferior vena cava
Middle lobe of right lung
Sinus venarum
Oblique fissure
Lower lobe of right lung
Pleural cavity
External intercostal m.
Internal intercostal m.
Innermost intercostal m.
Diaphragm
Liver
Serratus anterior m.
Latissimus dorsi m.
Esophagus
Azygos v.
Thoracic duct
Intercostal n.

Right coronary a.
Body of sternum

Cusps of tricuspid valve

Internal thoracic a. & v.

Right ventricle
Interventricular septum
Fifth rib
Anterior descending interventricular a.
Upper lobe of left lung
Oblique fissure
Lower lobe of left lung
Sixth rib
Wall of left ventricle
Seventh rib
Coronary sinus
Eighth rib
Descending aorta
Hemiazygos v.
Ninth rib
Thickened parietal pleura
Sympathetic ganglion
Body of the ninth thoracic vertebra
Transverse process of ninth thoracic vertebra
Spinous process of eighth thoracic vertebra
Spinal cord
Transversospinal m.
Trapezius m.
Sacrospinalis m.

The plane of section passes through the inferior mediastinum at the level of the lower border of the ninth thoracic vertebra and the dome of the diaphragm.

Transverse Section

THORAX.   Plate 3-16

Part IV

Abdomen

Plates 4-1 to 4-15

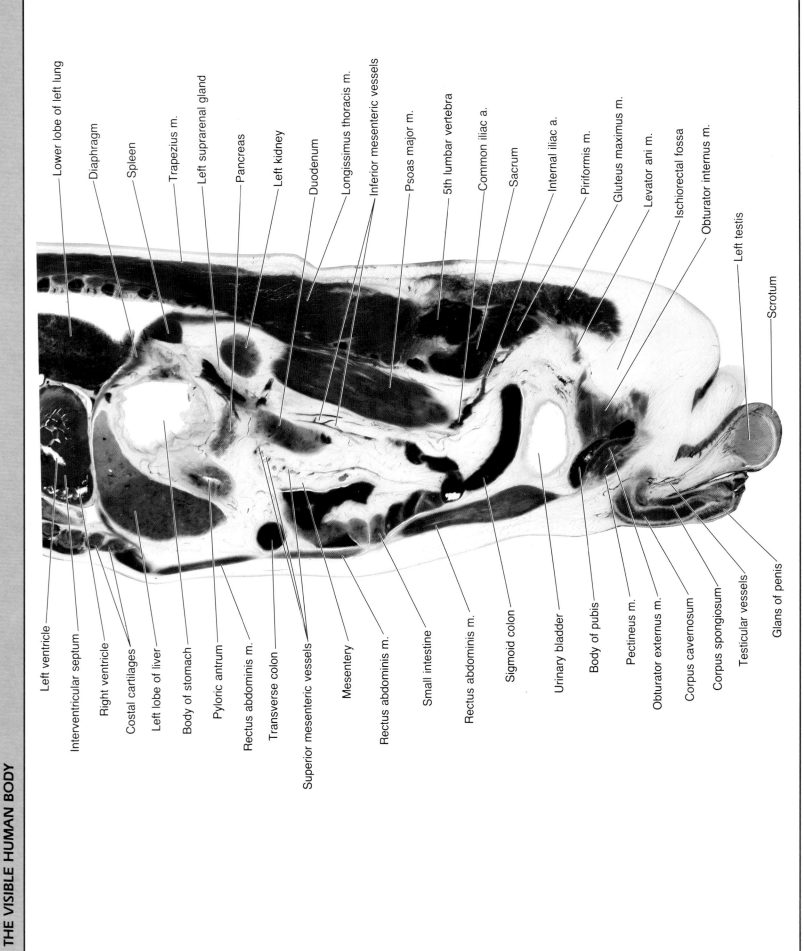

Left ventricle

Interventricular septum

Right ventricle

Costal cartilages

Left lobe of liver

Body of stomach

Pyloric antrum

Rectus abdominis m.

Transverse colon

Superior mesenteric vessels

Mesentery

Rectus abdominis m.

Small intestine

Rectus abdominis m.

Sigmoid colon

Urinary bladder

Body of pubis

Pectineus m.

Obturator externus m.

Corpus cavernosum

Corpus spongiosum

Testicular vessels

Glans of penis

Lower lobe of left lung

Diaphragm

Spleen

Trapezius m.

Left suprarenal gland

Pancreas

Left kidney

Duodenum

Longissimus thoracis m.

Inferior mesenteric vessels

Psoas major m.

5th lumbar vertebra

Common iliac a.

Sacrum

Internal iliac a.

Piriformis m.

Gluteus maximus m.

Levator ani m.

Ischiorectal fossa

Obturator internus m.

Left testis

Scrotum

Sagittal Section

The plane of section is slightly oblique. It passes to the left of the median plane — approximately 3 cm posteriorly and 1 cm anteriorly.

ABDOMEN.
Plate 4-1

Pectoralis major m

Upper lobe of left lung

Costal cartilages

Rectus abdominis m.

Diaphragm

Body of stomach

Peritoneal cavity

Transverse colon

Rectus abdominis m.

Tendinous intersection

Small intestine

Rectus abdominis m.

Mesentery

Rectus abdominis m.

Ilium

Internal abdominal oblique m.

Body of ischium

Head of femur

Femoral n.

Tendon of iliopsoas m.

Femoral a.

Femoral v.

Obturator externus m.

Lesser trochanter

Adductor longus m.

Adductor brevis m.

Adductor magnus m.

Oblique fissure

Lower lobe of left lung

Diaphragm

Latissimus dorsi m.

Spleen

Left kidney

Iliocostalis m.

Quadratus lumborum m.

Iliac crest

Iliacus m.

Gluteus medius m.

Superior gluteal vessels

Gluteus minimus m.

Piriformis m.

Gluteus maximus m.

Sciatic n.

Superior gemellus m.

Obturator internus m.

Inferior gemellus m.

Quadratus femoris m.

Sciatic n.

Biceps femoris m.

Semitendinosus m.

ABDOMEN.   Plate 4-2

The plane of section passes approximately 8 cm to the left of the median plane.

Sagittal Section

Apex of heart

Pericardial cavity

Body of sternum

Left lobe of liver

Hepatic v.

Right lobe of liver

Diaphragm

Middle lobe of right lung

Pleural cavity

Lower lobe of right lung

Innermost intercostal m.

Internal intercostal m.

External intercostal m.

Inferior vena cava

Caudate lobe of liver

Esophagus

Azygos v.

Serratus anterior m.

Latissimus dorsi m.

Posterior intercostal v.

Lymph node

Fifth rib

Sixth rib

Upper lobe of left lung

Thoracic duct

Lower lobe of left lung

Seventh rib

Aorta

Hemiazygos v.

Eighth rib

Intercostal n.

Ninth rib

Thickened parietal pleura

Tenth thoracic vertebra

Tenth rib

Costovertebral joint cavity

Spinal cord

Spinous process of ninth thoracic vertebra

Multifidus m.

Longissimus thoracis m.

Iliocostalis lumborum m.

Anterior longitudinal ligament

Section through the thoracoabdominal region passing through the upper border of the tenth thoracic vertebra. Liver, both lungs, and apex of the heart are included in the section.

Transverse Section

ABDOMEN.   Plate 4-3

Costal cartilages

Peritoneal cavity

Pericardial cavity

External abdominal oblique m.

Sixth rib

Upper lobe of left lung

Fundus of stomach

Cardia of stomach

Seventh rib

Thoracic duct

Aorta

Lower lobe of left lung

Eighth rib

Intercostal n.

Ninth rib

Hemiazygos v.

Thickened parietal pleura

Tenth thoracic vertebra

Tenth rib

Vertebral v.

Spinal cord

Left lobe of liver

Multifidus m.

Longissimus thoracis m.

Iliocostalis lumborum m.

Intercostal a.

Latissimus dorsi m.

Lower lobe of right lung

Serratus anterior m.

Azygos v.

Caudate lobe of liver

Inferior vena cava

Hepatic v.

External intercostal m.

Internal intercostal m.

Innermost intercostal m.

Pleural cavity

Diaphragm

Middle lobe of right lung

Right lobe of liver

Quadrate lobe of liver

Falciform ligament

Section through the thoracoabdominal region passing through the lower border of the tenth thoracic vertebra. Liver and fundus of the stomach are included in the section.

ABDOMEN.   Plate 4-4

Transverse Section

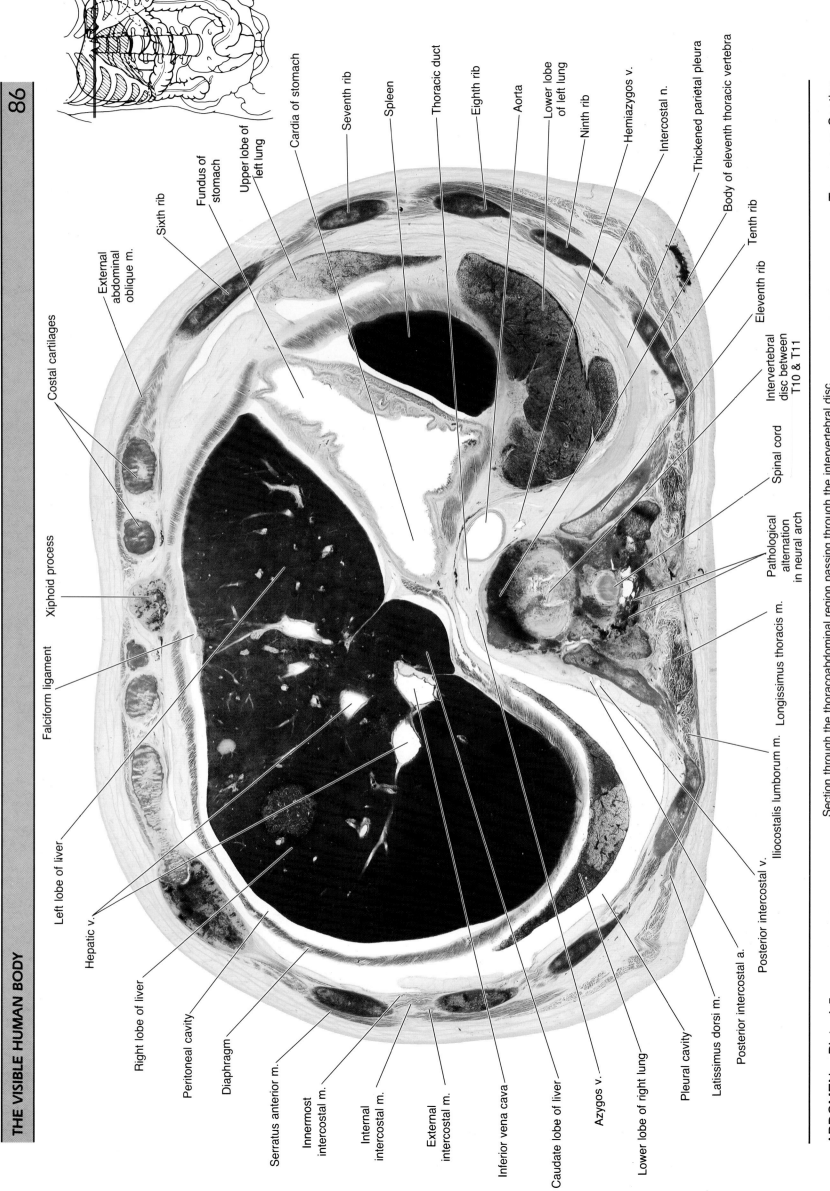

Costal cartilages

External
abdominal
oblique m.

Sixth rib

Fundus of
stomach

Upper lobe of
left lung

Cardia of stomach

Seventh rib

Spleen

Thoracic duct

Eighth rib

Aorta

Lower lobe
of left lung

Ninth rib

Hemiazygos v.

Intercostal n.

Thickened parietal pleura

Body of eleventh thoracic vertebra

Tenth rib

Eleventh rib

Intervertebral
disc between
T10 & T11

Spinal cord

Pathological
alternation
in neural arch

Longissimus thoracis m.

Iliocostalis lumborum m.

Posterior intercostal v.

Posterior intercostal a.

Latissimus dorsi m.

Pleural cavity

Lower lobe of right lung

Azygos v.

Inferior vena cava

Caudate lobe of liver

External
intercostal m.

Internal
intercostal m.

Innermost
intercostal m.

Serratus anterior m.

Diaphragm

Peritoneal cavity

Right lobe of liver

Hepatic v.

Left lobe of liver

Falciform ligament

Xiphoid process

Section through the thoracoabdominal region passing through the intervertebral disc
between T10 & T11. Liver, stomach, and spleen are included in the section.

Transverse Section

ABDOMEN. Plate 4-5

Rectus abdominis m.

Costal cartilages

Hepatogastric ligament

Sixth rib

External abdominal oblique m.

Body of stomach

Lesser omentum

Upper lobe of left lung

Seventh rib

Costodiaphragmatic recess

Left gastric a.

Thoracic duct

Eighth rib

Aorta

Spleen

Ninth rib

Inferior phrenic a.

Hemiazygos v.

Posterior intercostal v.

Tenth rib

Thickened parietal pleura

Eleventh rib

Pathological fusion of T11 & T12 vertebra

Left lobe of liver

Xiphoid process

Falciform ligament

Right lobe of liver

Hepatic triad

Diaphragm

Pleural cavity

Peritoneal cavity

Serratus anterior m.

Hepatic v.

Inferior vena cava

Caudate lobe of liver

Azygos v.

Latissimus dorsi m.

Iliocostalis lumborum m.

Longissimus thoracis m.

Pathological alteration in neural arch

Spinal cord

Transverse Section

Section through the thoracoabdominal region passing through the eleventh thoracic vertebra. Liver, body of the stomach, and spleen are included in the section.

ABDOMEN.   Plate 4-6

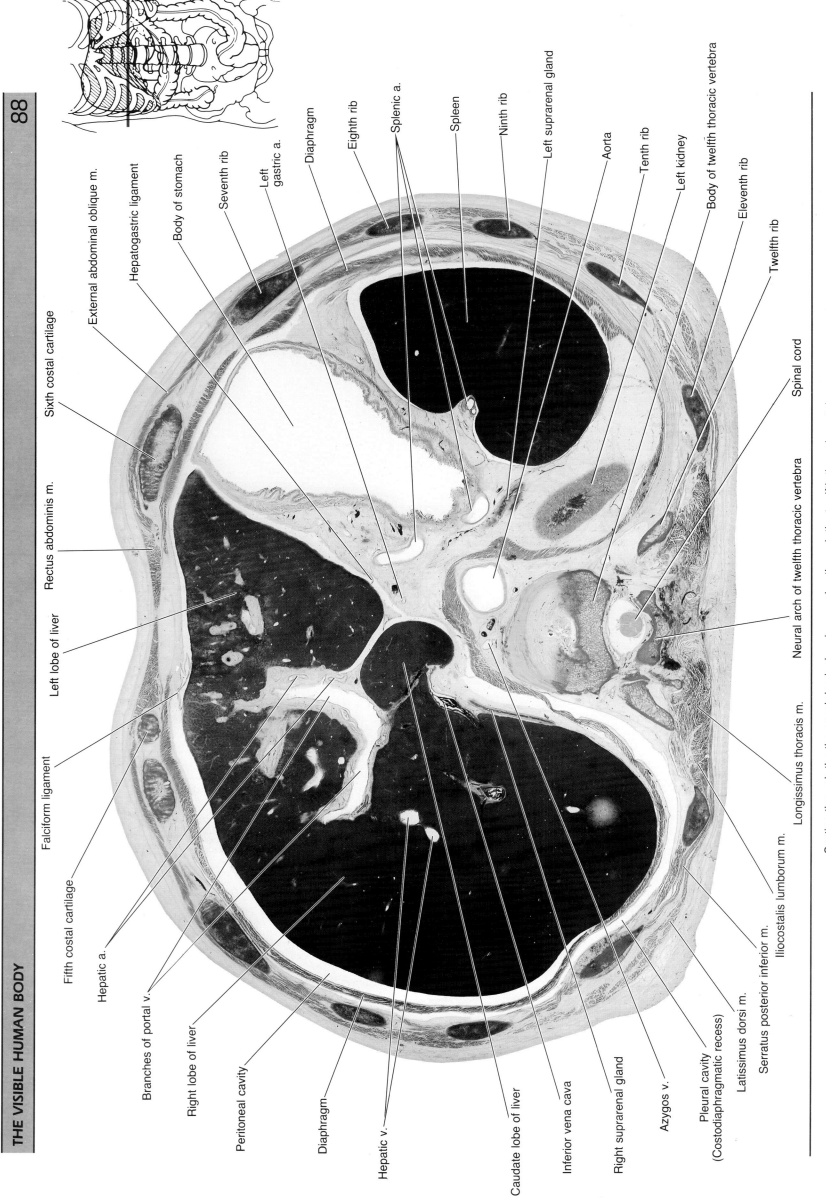

Falciform ligament

Sixth costal cartilage

External abdominal oblique m.

Hepatogastric ligament

Body of stomach

Seventh rib

Left gastric a.

Diaphragm

Eighth rib

Splenic a.

Spleen

Ninth rib

Left suprarenal gland

Aorta

Tenth rib

Left kidney

Body of twelfth thoracic vertebra

Eleventh rib

Twelfth rib

Rectus abdominis m.

Fifth costal cartilage

Hepatic a.

Branches of portal v.

Right lobe of liver

Peritoneal cavity

Left lobe of liver

Diaphragm

Hepatic v.

Caudate lobe of liver

Inferior vena cava

Right suprarenal gland

Azygos v.

Pleural cavity
(Costodiaphragmatic recess)

Latissimus dorsi m.

Serratus posterior inferior m.

Iliocostalis lumborum m.

Longissimus thoracis m.

Neural arch of twelfth thoracic vertebra

Spinal cord

Section through the thoracoabdominal region passing through the twelfth thoracic vertebra.
Left kidney, both suprarenal glands, and splenic artery are included in the section.

ABDOMEN.   Plate 4-7   Transverse Section

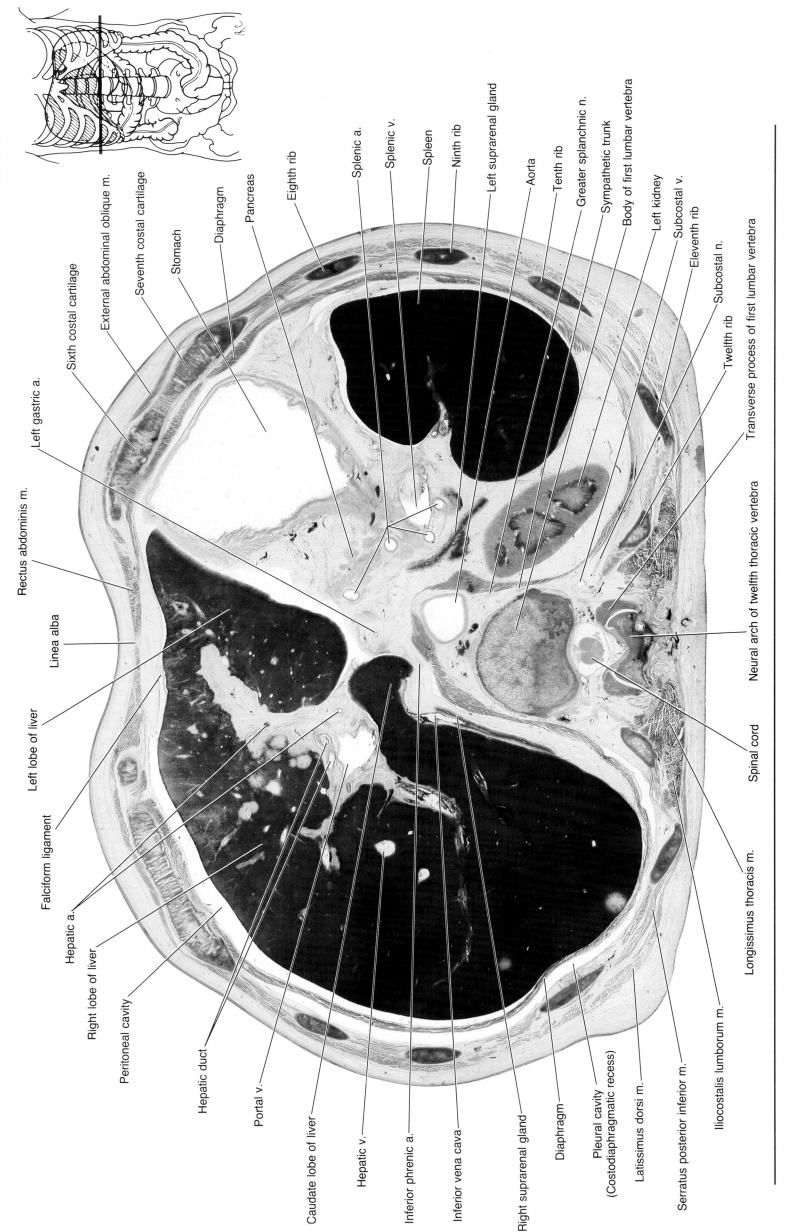

Rectus abdominis m.

Left gastric a.

Sixth costal cartilage

External abdominal oblique m.

Seventh costal cartilage

Stomach

Diaphragm

Pancreas

Eighth rib

Splenic a.

Splenic v.

Spleen

Ninth rib

Left suprarenal gland

Aorta

Tenth rib

Greater splanchnic n.

Sympathetic trunk

Body of first lumbar vertebra

Left kidney

Subcostal v.

Eleventh rib

Subcostal n.

Twelfth rib

Transverse process of first lumbar vertebra

Linea alba

Left lobe of liver

Falciform ligament

Hepatic a.

Right lobe of liver

Peritoneal cavity

Hepatic duct

Portal v.

Caudate lobe of liver

Hepatic v.

Inferior phrenic a.

Inferior vena cava

Right suprarenal gland

Diaphragm

Pleural cavity
(Costodiaphragmatic recess)

Latissimus dorsi m.

Serratus posterior inferior m.

Iliocostalis lumborum m.

Longissimus thoracis m.

Spinal cord

Neural arch of twelfth thoracic vertebra

Section through the thoracoabdominal region passing through the first lumbar vertebra.
The body of the pancreas and splenic artery are included in the section.

Transverse Section

ABDOMEN.   Plate 4-8

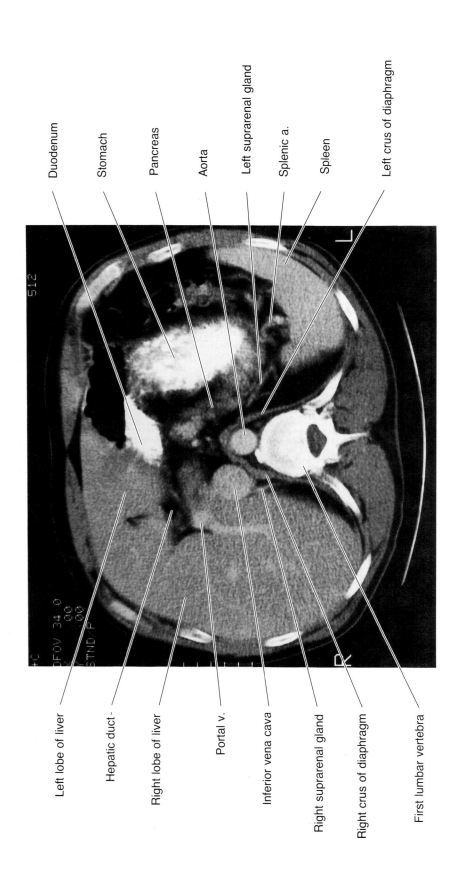

Duodenum

Stomach

Pancreas

Aorta

Left suprarenal gland

Splenic a.

Spleen

Left crus of diaphragm

Left lobe of liver

Hepatic duct-

Right lobe of liver

Portal v.

Inferior vena cava

Right suprarenal gland

Right crus of diaphragm

First lumbar vertebra

The sections shown in Plate 4-9 and the accompanying CT (Plate 4-9 CT) pass in a transverse plane through the abdomen at the level of the first lumbar vertebra. However, the plane in Plate 4-9 CT passes through the abdomen slightly above the plane of the section in Plate 4-9; therefore it is helpful to also compare Plate 4-9 CT with Plate 4-8. In Plate 4-9, some of the organs that border the lesser sac can be seen. These include the stomach, pancreas, and spleen. (Various relationships of the structures that border the lesser sac can be studied in Plates 4-1 through 4-12.) The splenic artery and vein can be seen as they lie posterior to the body of the pancreas and pass to the hilum of the spleen. Both the left and right suprarenal glands can be identified in the section. The right suprarenal lies adjacent to the right lobe of the liver. The left suprarenal lies adjacent to the superior aspect of the left kidney. In the accompanying CT, the section is at a slightly superior level and does not include the left kidney. In the CT, the stomach, pancreas, spleen, splenic artery, liver, and both suprarenal glands are clearly visible. Note that in the CT the stomach and duodenum appear as the structures with the most contrast. This is due to the use of a barium solution as a medium to enhance contrast in order to facilitate the viewing of components of the gastrointestinal tract.

In both plates, the aorta can be seen as it lies between the crura of the diaphragm. In Plate 4-9 the section includes the celiac trunk and two of the arteries that arise from it, namely the common hepatic and splenic arteries. To the right of the aorta, the inferior vena cava lies adjacent to the liver in the caval groove. The caudate lobe of the liver separates the inferior vena cava from the porta hepatis, located between the quadrate and caudate lobes of the liver. At the porta hepatis the portal vein and hepatic artery with its associated autonomic nerve plexus enter the liver and the hepatic ducts and lymphatic vessels emerge from it. In both plates, the portal vein and hepatic duct are identified in the porta hepatis. Due to the absence of blood and the pressure produced by the weight of the overlying liver in the cadaver used to obtain this series of specimens, the inferior vena cava appears flattened in Plates 4-7 to 4-15. In the Plate 4-9 CT, the normal anatomy of the inferior vena cava is maintained.

The large tumors seen in the quadrate lobe of the liver in Plate 4-9 are due to the presence of a metastatic malignant melanoma (see Plate 3-13 CT).

Plate 4-9 CT
Transverse Section

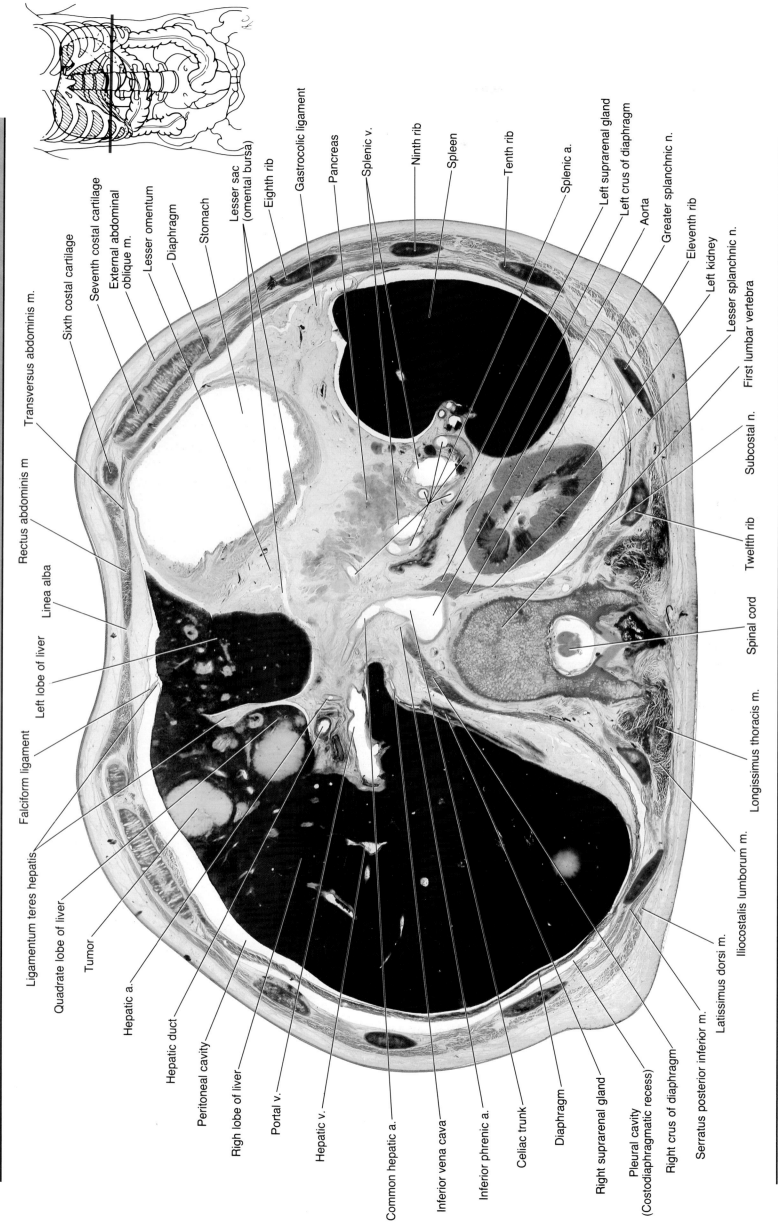

Ligamentum teres hepatis

Falciform ligament

Rectus abdominis m.

Transversus abdominis m.

Sixth costal cartilage

Seventh costal cartilage

External abdominal oblique m.

Lesser omentum

Diaphragm

Stomach

Lesser sac (omental bursa)

Eighth rib

Gastrocolic ligament

Pancreas

Splenic v.

Ninth rib

Spleen

Tenth rib

Splenic a.

Left suprarenal gland

Left crus of diaphragm

Aorta

Greater splanchnic n.

Eleventh rib

Left kidney

Lesser splanchnic n.

First lumbar vertebra

Quadrate lobe of liver

Tumor

Hepatic a.

Linea alba

Left lobe of liver

Hepatic duct

Peritoneal cavity

Righ lobe of liver

Portal v.

Hepatic v.

Common hepatic a.

Inferior vena cava

Inferior phrenic a.

Celiac trunk

Diaphragm

Right suprarenal gland

Pleural cavity (Costodiaphragmatic recess)

Right crus of diaphragm

Serratus posterior inferior m.

Latissimus dorsi m.

Iliocostalis lumborum m.

Longissimus thoracis m.

Spinal cord

Twelfth rib

Subcostal n.

ABDOMEN.   Plate 4-9

Transverse Section

Section through the thoracoabdominal region passing through the first lumbar vertebra.
The body of the pancreas, splenic artery, and celiac trunk are included in the section.

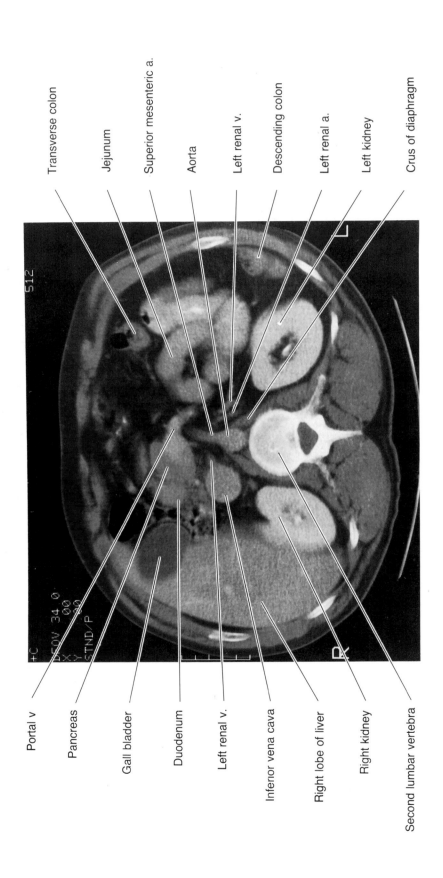

Transverse colon

Jejunum

Superior mesenteric a.

Aorta

Left renal v.

Descending colon

Left renal a.

Left kidney

Crus of diaphragm

Portal v

Pancreas

Gall bladder

Duodenum

Left renal v.

Inferior vena cava

Right lobe of liver

Right kidney

Second lumbar vertebra

The sections shown in Plate 4-10 and 4-11 and the accompanying CT (Plate 4-10 CT) pass in a transverse plane through the abdomen at the level of the second lumbar vertebra. The superior mesenteric artery is identified in Plates 4-10 and 4-10 CT as it arises from the aorta. However, the plane in Plate 4-10 CT passes through the abdomen slightly below the plane of the section in Plate 4-10; therefore, it is helpful to also compare Plate 4-10 CT with Plate 4-11. As we explained in the legend for Plate 4-9, the relationships of structures that border the lesser sac can be studied in Plates 4-1 through 4-12. In Plates 4-10 and 4-11, portions of the stomach, pancreas, spleen, and gall bladder can be seen. The section shown in Plate 4-10 includes the gall bladder, cystic and hepatic ducts, hepatic artery, pyloric antrum, and portions of the body and tail of the pancreas. In this plate the splenic artery and vein are seen as they pass along the posterior surface of the body of the pancreas to reach the hilum of the spleen (see also Plate 4-9). The pyloric antrum and sphincter, first part of the duodenum, and head of the pancreas are included in Plate 4-11. The common bile duct, portal vein, and gastroduodenal artery can be seen in association with the head of the pancreas. Plate 4-10 CT includes the head of the pancreas and demonstrates the relationship of the portal vein

to this portion of the pancreas (compare with Plate 4-11); however the section does not include the spleen. The presence of the spleen in Plates 4-10 and 4-11 is due to is abnormally large size.

In Plate 4-10 both the left and right suprarenal glands can be identified in the section; in Plate 4-11 they are not present but both kidneys are included in the section. As was explained in the legend for Plate 4-9, the inferior vena cava is flattened. In Plate 4-11 the left renal vein can be seen as it extends from the inferior vena cava across the anterior surface of the aorta to reach the hilum of the left kidney. The left renal artery is seen as it lies posterior to the left renal vein. A portion of the left renal pelvis is also included in the section. In Plate 4-10 CT, the section is at a slightly superior level to that of Plate 4-11 and does not include the portion of the left renal vein that crosses anterior to the aorta; however the proximal and distal portions of the renal vein are visible. The CT also includes portions of the left renal artery.

The tumors seen in the liver in Plates 4-10 and 4-11 are due to the presence of a metastatic malignant melanoma (see Plate 3-13 CT).

Plate 4-10 CT
Transverse Section

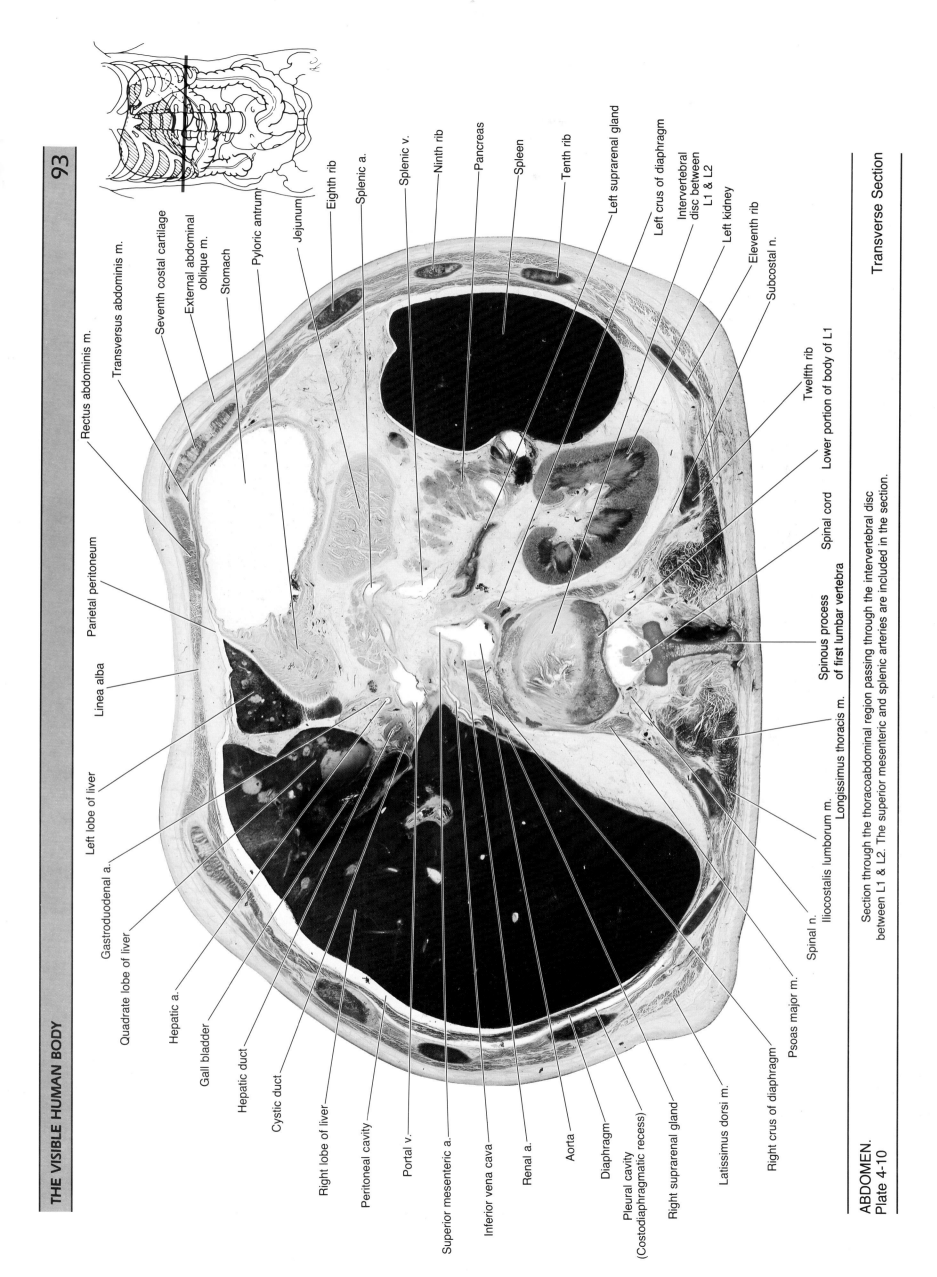

Rectus abdominis m.

Transversus abdominis m.

Seventh costal cartilage

External abdominal oblique m.

Stomach

Pyloric antrum

Jejunum

Eighth rib

Splenic a.

Splenic v.

Ninth rib

Pancreas

Spleen

Tenth rib

Left suprarenal gland

Left crus of diaphragm

Intervertebral disc between L1 & L2

Left kidney

Eleventh rib

Subcostal n.

Twelfth rib

Lower portion of body of L1

Spinous process of first lumbar vertebra

Spinal cord

Parietal peritoneum

Linea alba

Left lobe of liver

Gastroduodenal a.

Quadrate lobe of liver

Hepatic a.

Gall bladder

Hepatic duct

Cystic duct

Right lobe of liver

Peritoneal cavity

Portal v.

Superior mesenteric a.

Inferior vena cava

Renal a.

Aorta

Diaphragm

Pleural cavity (Costodiaphragmatic recess)

Right suprarenal gland

Latissimus dorsi m.

Right crus of diaphragm

Psoas major m.

Spinal n.

Iliocostalis lumborum m.

Longissimus thoracis m.

Section through the thoracoabdominal region passing through the intervertebral disc between L1 & L2. The superior mesenteric and splenic arteries are included in the section.

Transverse Section

ABDOMEN.
Plate 4-10

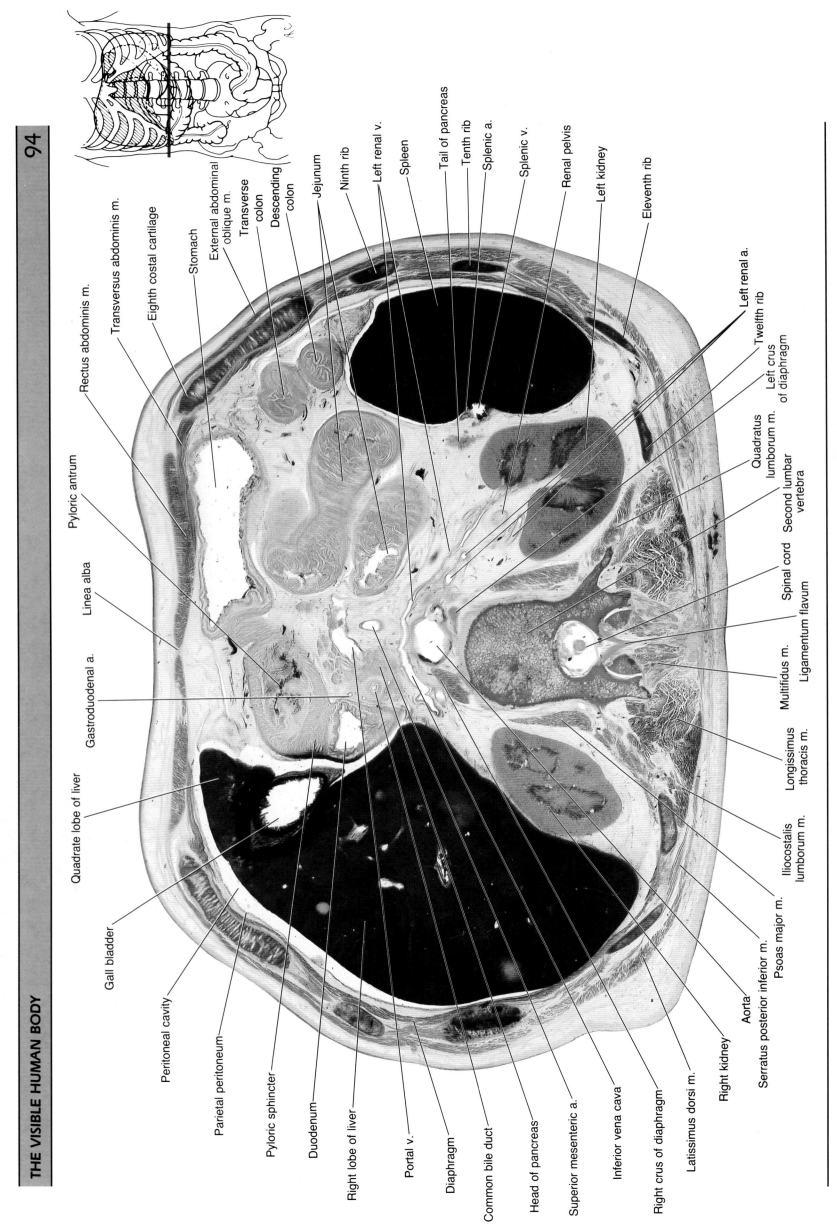

Rectus abdominis m.

Transversus abdominis m.

Eighth costal cartilage

Stomach

External abdominal oblique m.

Transverse colon

Descending colon

Jejunum

Ninth rib

Left renal v.

Spleen

Tail of pancreas

Tenth rib

Splenic a.

Splenic v.

Renal pelvis

Left kidney

Eleventh rib

Left renal a.

Twelfth rib

Left crus of diaphragm

Quadratus lumborum m.

Second lumbar vertebra

Spinal cord

Ligamentum flavum

Multifidus m.

Longissimus thoracis m.

Iliocostalis lumborum m.

Psoas major m.

Serratus posterior inferior m.

Aorta

Right kidney

Latissimus dorsi m.

Right crus of diaphragm

Inferior vena cava

Superior mesenteric a.

Head of pancreas

Common bile duct

Diaphragm

Portal v.

Right lobe of liver

Duodenum

Pyloric sphincter

Peritoneal cavity

Parietal peritoneum

Gall bladder

Quadrate lobe of liver

Gastroduodenal a.

Linea alba

Pyloric antrum

Section through the abdomen passing through the second lumbar vertebra. Gall bladder, pyloric sphincter, left renal artery and vein, and both kidneys are included in the section.

Transverse Section

ABDOMEN.   Plate 4-11

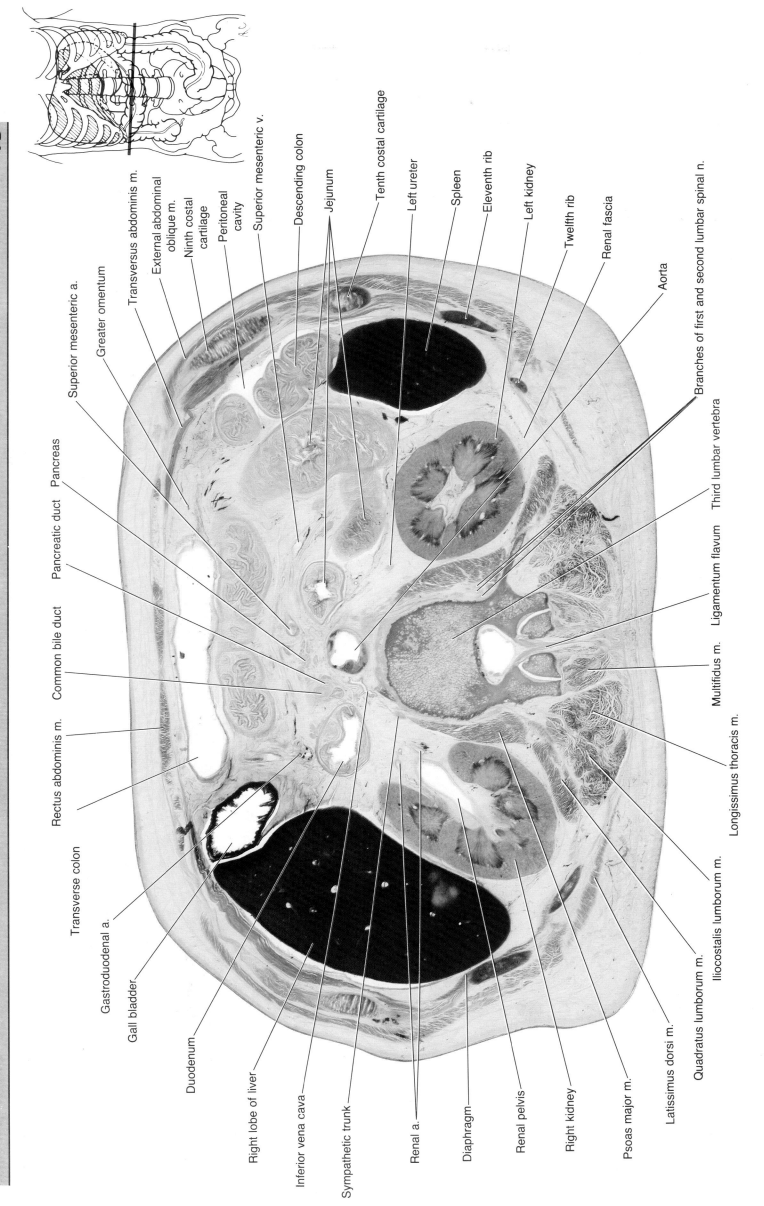

Superior mesenteric a.

Greater omentum

Transversus abdominis m.

External abdominal oblique m.

Ninth costal cartilage

Peritoneal cavity

Superior mesenteric v.

Descending colon

Jejunum

Tenth costal cartilage

Left ureter

Spleen

Eleventh rib

Left kidney

Twelfth rib

Renal fascia

Aorta

Branches of first and second lumbar spinal n.

Third lumbar vertebra

Ligamentum flavum

Multifidus m.

Longissimus thoracis m.

Iliocostalis lumborum m.

Quadratus lumborum m.

Latissimus dorsi m.

Psoas major m.

Right kidney

Renal pelvis

Diaphragm

Renal a.

Sympathetic trunk

Inferior vena cava

Right lobe of liver

Duodenum

Gall bladder

Gastroduodenal a.

Transverse colon

Rectus abdominis m.

Common bile duct

Pancreatic duct

Pancreas

Section through the abdomen passing through the third lumbar vertebra. Transverse colon, common bile duct, pancreatic duct, gall bladder, and kidneys are included in the section.

Transverse Section

ABDOMEN.   Plate 4-12

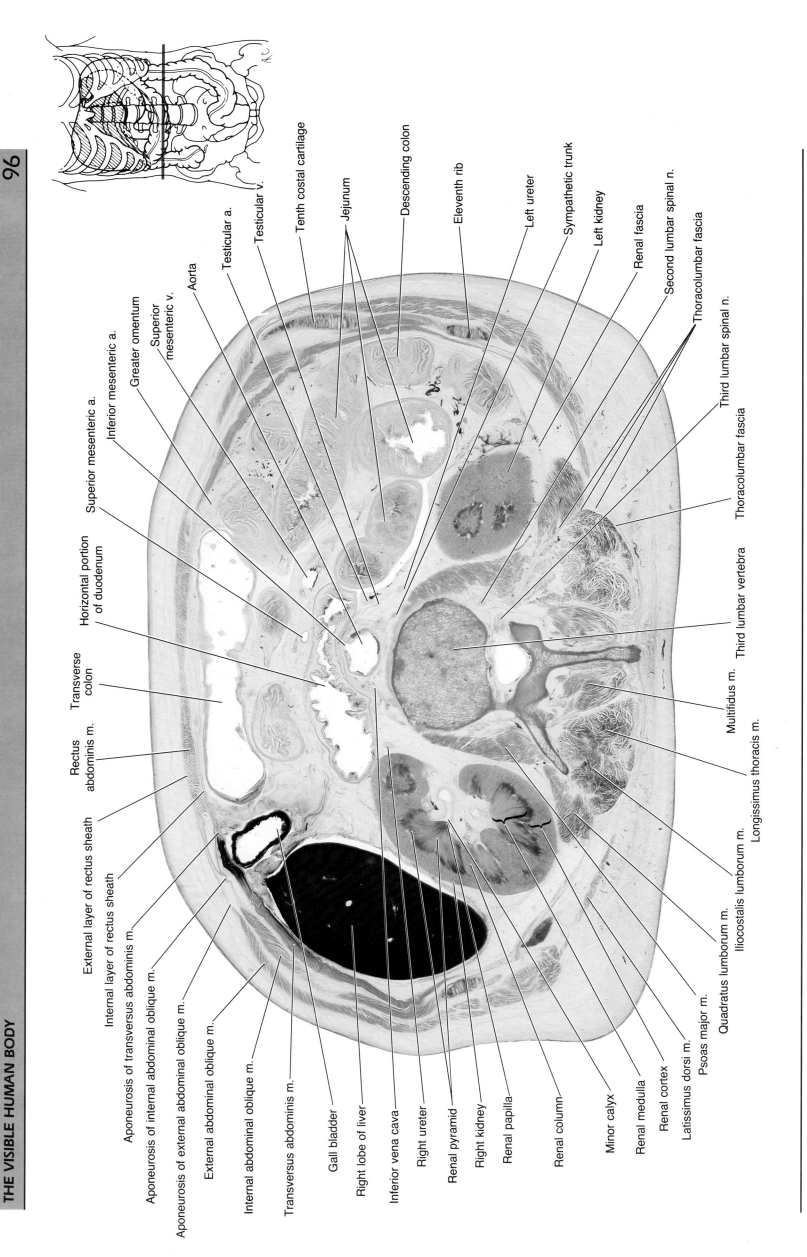

Superior mesenteric a.

Inferior mesenteric a.

Greater omentum

Superior mesenteric v.

Aorta

Testicular a.

Testicular v.

Tenth costal cartilage

Jejunum

Descending colon

Eleventh rib

Left ureter

Sympathetic trunk

Left kidney

Renal fascia

Second lumbar spinal n.

Thoracolumbar fascia

Third lumbar spinal n.

External layer of rectus sheath

Internal layer of rectus sheath

Aponeurosis of transversus abdominis m.

Aponeurosis of internal abdominal oblique m.

External abdominal oblique m.

Aponeurosis of external abdominal oblique m.

Internal abdominal oblique m.

Transversus abdominis m.

Gall bladder

Right lobe of liver

Inferior vena cava

Right ureter

Renal pyramid

Right kidney

Renal papilla

Rectus abdominis m.

Transverse colon

Horizontal portion of duodenum

Renal column

Minor calyx

Renal medulla

Renal cortex

Latissimus dorsi m.

Psoas major m.

Quadratus lumborum m.

Iliocostalis lumborum m.

Longissimus thoracis m.

Multifidus m.

Third lumbar vertebra

Thoracolumbar fascia

ABDOMEN.   Plate 4-13

Transverse Section

Section through the abdomen passing through the lower border of the third lumbar
vertebra. The horizontal portion of the duodenum is included in the section.

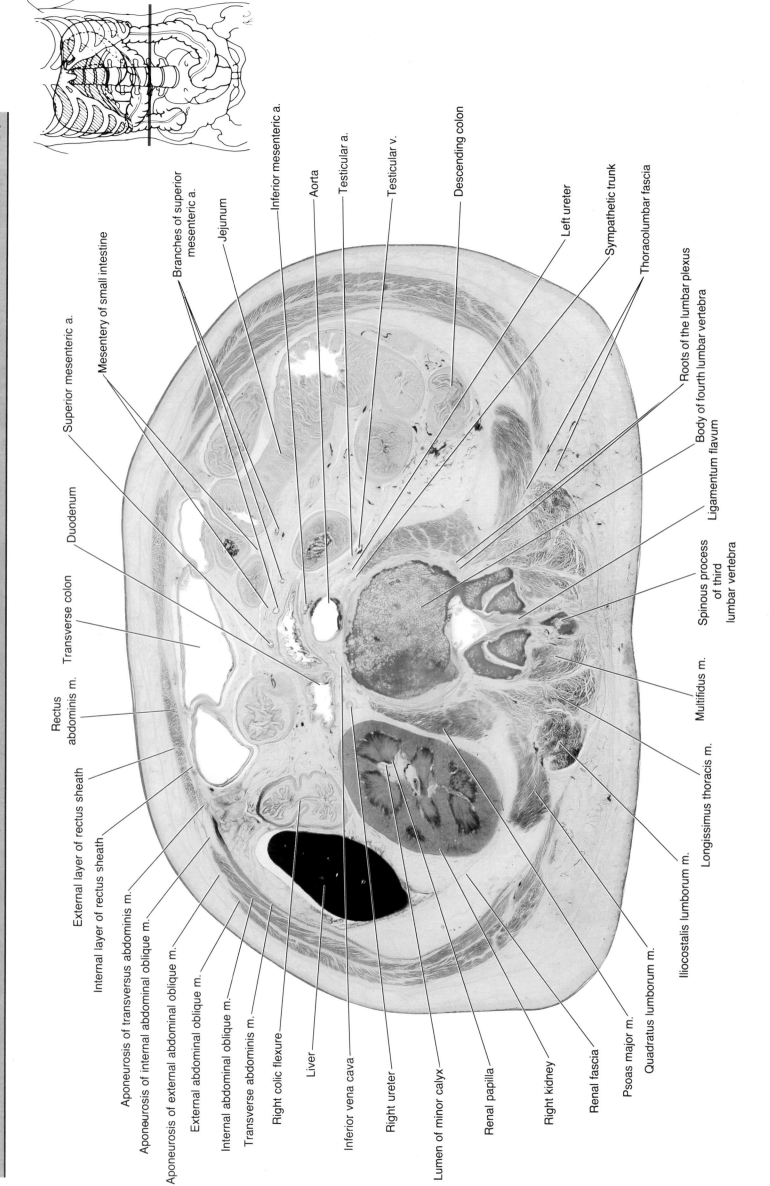

Mesentery of small intestine

Branches of superior
mesenteric a.

Jejunum

Inferior mesenteric a.

Aorta

Testicular a.

Testicular v.

Descending colon

Left ureter

Sympathetic trunk

Thoracolumbar fascia

Roots of the lumbar plexus

Body of fourth lumbar vertebra

Ligamentum flavum

Spinous process
of third
lumbar vertebra

Multifidus m.

Longissimus thoracis m.

Iliocostalis lumborum m.

Quadratus lumborum m.

Psoas major m.

Renal fascia

Right kidney

Renal papilla

Lumen of minor calyx

Right ureter

Inferior vena cava

Liver

Right colic flexure

Transverse abdominis m.

Internal abdominal oblique m.

External abdominal oblique m.

Aponeurosis of external abdominal oblique m.

Aponeurosis of internal abdominal oblique m.

Aponeurosis of transversus abdominis m.

Internal layer of rectus sheath

External layer of rectus sheath

Rectus
abdominis m.

Transverse colon

Duodenum

Superior mesenteric a.

ABDOMEN.   Plate 4-14

Section through the abdomen passing through the fourth lumbar vertebra. Right kidney,
right colic flexure, and lower border of the duodenum are included in the section.

Transverse Section

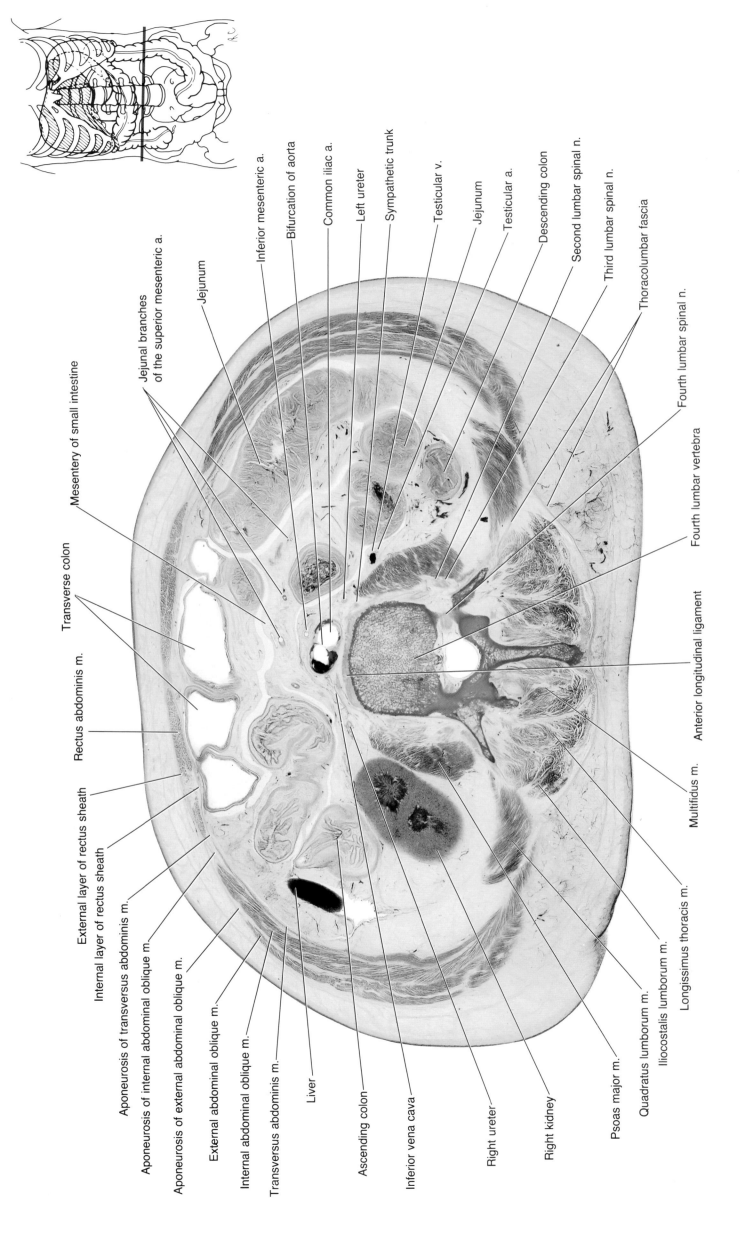

External layer of rectus sheath

Internal layer of rectus sheath

Aponeurosis of transversus abdominis m.

Aponeurosis of internal abdominal oblique m.

Aponeurosis of external abdominal oblique m.

External abdominal oblique m.

Internal abdominal oblique m.

Transversus abdominis m.

Liver

Ascending colon

Inferior vena cava

Right ureter

Right kidney

Psoas major m.

Quadratus lumborum m.

Iliocostalis lumborum m.

Longissimus thoracis m.

Multifidus m.

Anterior longitudinal ligament

Fourth lumbar vertebra

Rectus abdominis m.

Transverse colon

Mesentery of small intestine

Jejunal branches
of the superior mesenteric a.

Jejunum

Inferior mesenteric a.

Bifurcation of aorta

Common iliac a.

Left ureter

Sympathetic trunk

Testicular v.

Jejunum

Testicular a.

Descending colon

Second lumbar spinal n.

Third lumbar spinal n.

Thoracolumbar fascia

Fourth lumbar spinal n.

ABDOMEN.   Plate 4-15

Section through the abdomen passing through the fourth lumbar vertebra. The bifurcation
of the aorta, transverse colon, and lower pole of the right kidney are included in the section.

Transverse Section

Part V

Male Pelvis and Perineum

Plates 5-1 to 5-13

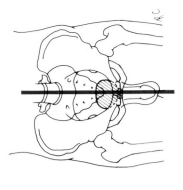

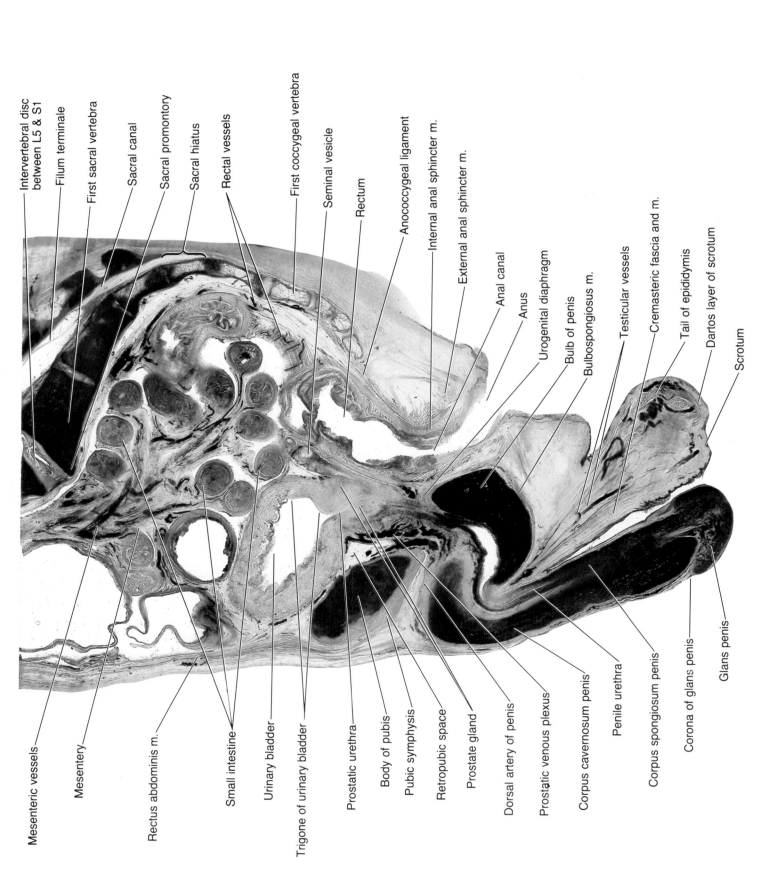

Mesenteric vessels

Mesentery

Rectus abdominis m.

Small intestine

Urinary bladder

Trigone of urinary bladder

Prostatic urethra

Body of pubis

Pubic symphysis

Retropubic space

Prostate gland

Dorsal artery of penis

Prostatic venous plexus

Corpus cavernosum penis

Penile urethra

Corpus spongiosum penis

Corona of glans penis

Glans penis

Intervertebral disc between L5 & S1

Filum terminale

First sacral vertebra

Sacral canal

Sacral promontory

Sacral hiatus

Rectal vessels

First coccygeal vertebra

Seminal vesicle

Rectum

Anococcygeal ligament

Internal anal sphincter m.

External anal sphincter m.

Anal canal

Anus

Urogenital diaphragm

Bulb of penis

Bulbospongiosus m.

Testicular vessels

Cremasteric fascia and m.

Tail of epididymis

Dartos layer of scrotum

Scrotum

MALE PELVIS AND
PERINEUM.   Plate 5-1

Sagittal Section

Section passes through the median plane. Bladder, prostate, seminal vesicle, rectum, urethra, and external genitalia are included in the section.

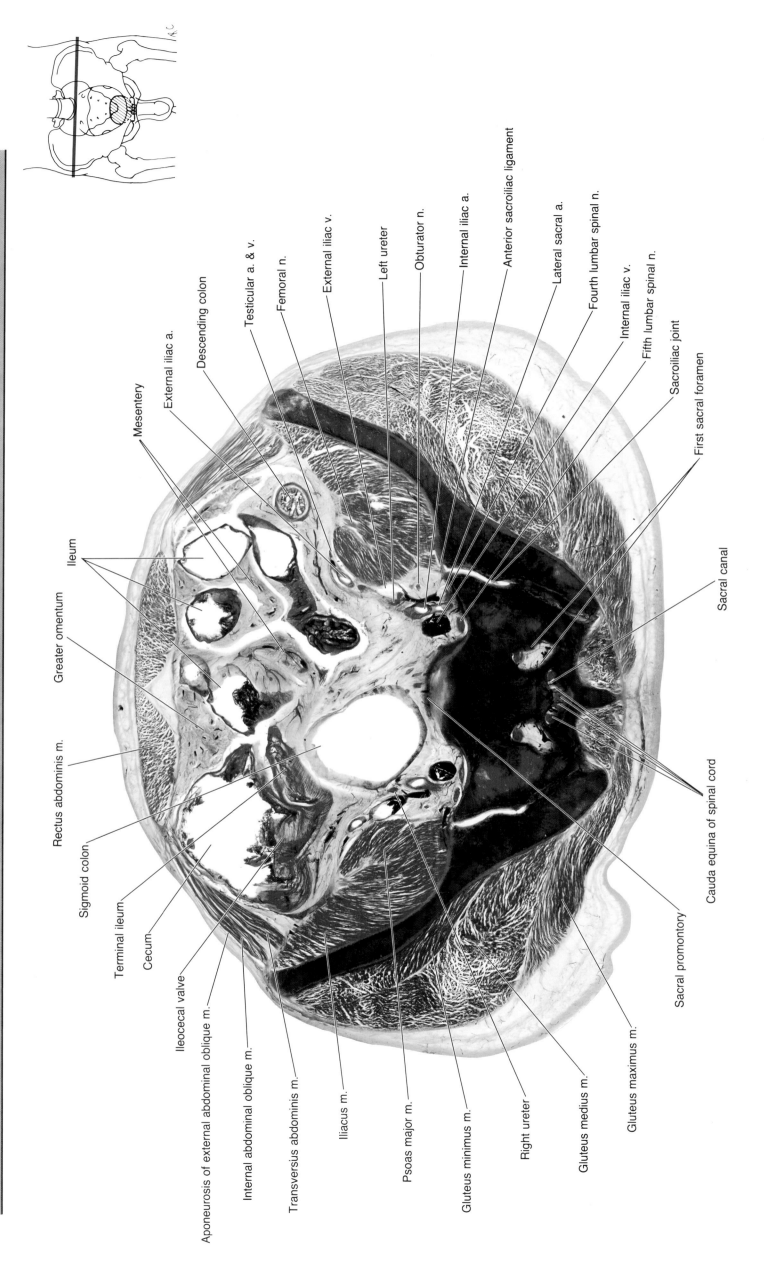

Mesentery

External iliac a.

Descending colon

Testicular a. & v.

Femoral n.

External iliac v.

Left ureter

Obturator n.

Internal iliac a.

Anterior sacroiliac ligament

Lateral sacral a.

Fourth lumbar spinal n.

Internal iliac v.

Fifth lumbar spinal n.

Sacroiliac joint

First sacral foramen

Sacral canal

Ileum

Greater omentum

Rectus abdominis m.

Sigmoid colon

Terminal ileum

Cecum

Ileocecal valve

Aponeurosis of external abdominal oblique m.

Internal abdominal oblique m.

Transversus abdominis m.

Iliacus m.

Psoas major m.

Gluteus minimus m.

Right ureter

Gluteus medius m.

Gluteus maximus m.

Sacral promontory

Cauda equina of spinal cord

MALE PELVIS AND
PERINEUM.   Plate 5-2

Section through the false pelvis at the level of the anterosuperior iliac spines and sacral
promontory. Cecum, ileocecal valve, and sigmoid colon are included in the section.

Transverse Section

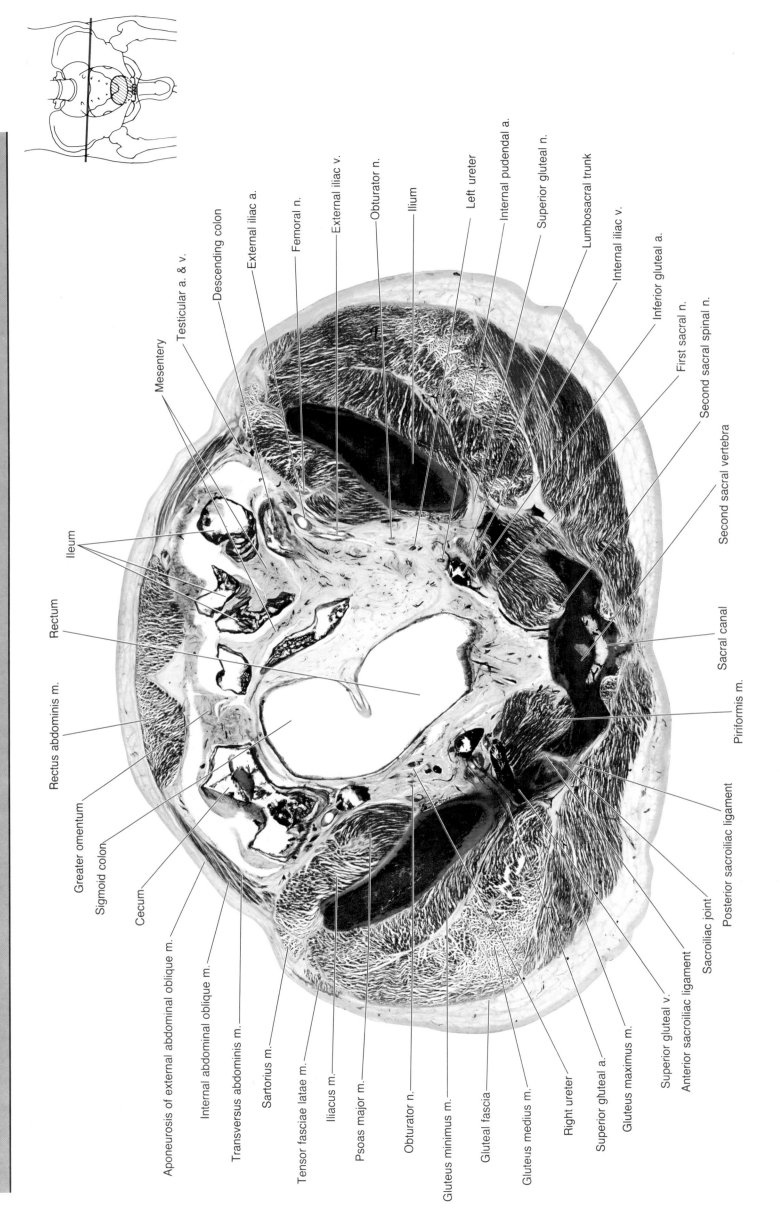

Aponeurosis of external abdominal oblique m.

Internal abdominal oblique m.

Transversus abdominis m.

Sartorius m.

Tensor fasciae latae m.

Iliacus m.

Psoas major m.

Obturator n.

Gluteus minimus m.

Gluteal fascia

Gluteus medius m.

Right ureter

Superior gluteal a.

Gluteus maximus m.

Superior gluteal v.

Anterior sacroiliac ligament

Sacroiliac joint

Posterior sacroiliac ligament

Piriformis m.

Sacral canal

Second sacral vertebra

Second sacral spinal n.

First sacral n.

Inferior gluteal a.

Internal iliac v.

Lumbosacral trunk

Superior gluteal n.

Internal pudendal a.

Left ureter

Ilium

Obturator n.

External iliac v.

Femoral n.

External iliac a.

Descending colon

Testicular a. & v.

Mesentery

Ileum

Rectum

Rectus abdominis m.

Greater omentum

Sigmoid colon

Cecum

MALE PELVIS AND
PERINEUM. Plate 5-3

Transverse Section

Section through the false pelvis passing approximately 2 cm below the anterosuperior iliac spines. Cecum, rectum, and superior gluteal artery and vein are included in the section.

Rectus abdominis m.

Greater omentum

Transversalis fascia

Cecum

Internal abdominal oblique m.

Rectum

Iliacus m.

Sartorius m.

Tensor fasciae latae m.

Psoas major m.

Gluteus minimus m.

Gluteus medius m.

Gluteal fascia

Obturator internus m.

Sigmoid colon

Ileum

Fermoral n.

External iliac a.

External iliac v.

Vas deferens

Obturator n.

Ilium

Deep branch of superior gluteal a. & v.

Left ureter

Internal pudendal a.

Internal iliac v.

Sacral plexus

Inferior gluteal v.

Inferior gluteal a.

Third sacral vertebra

Sacral canal

Internal iliac v.

Piriformis m.

Right ureter

Gluteus maximus m.

MALE PELVIS AND
PERINEUM. Plate 5-4

Transverse Section

Section through the false pelvis passing approximately 4 cm below the anterosuperior iliac spines. Cecum, sigmoid colon, and rectum are included in the section.

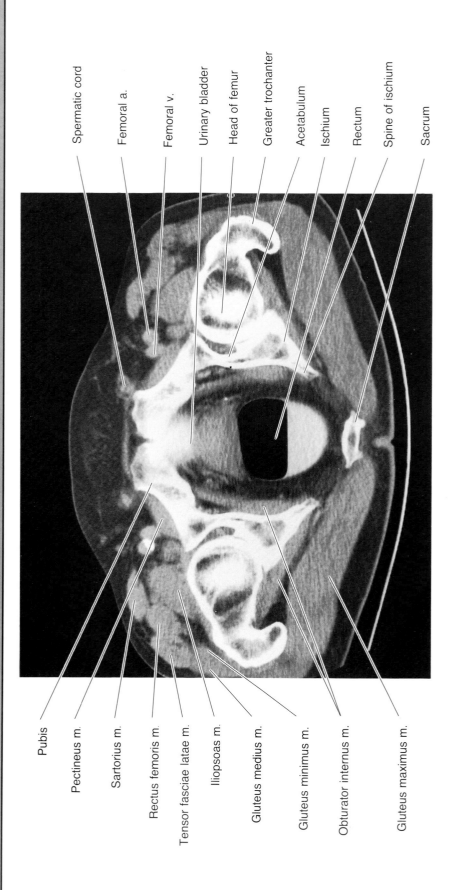

Pubis

Pectineus m.

Sartorius m.

Rectus femoris m.

Tensor fasciae latae m.

Iliopsoas m.

Gluteus medius m.

Gluteus minimus m.

Obturator internus m.

Gluteus maximus m.

Spermatic cord

Femoral a.

Femoral v.

Urinary bladder

Head of femur

Greater trochanter

Acetabulum

Ischium

Rectum

Spine of ischium

Sacrum

The sections shown in Plates 5-5 and 5-6 and the accompanying CT (Plate 5-5 CT) pass in transverse planes through the pelvis and head of the femur at the level of of the acetabulum. However, the sections in Plates 5-5 and 5-6, as compared with 5-5 CT, are at a slightly more superior level and are slightly oblique as they pass from anterior to posterior (the anterior border of the cut being slightly more superior as compared to the CT). Therefore, it is helpful to compare both of these plates with the CT.

The pelvic diaphragm, composed of the levator ani and coccygeus muscles, divides the cavity of the true pelvis into the main pelvic cavity above and the perineum below. In the main pelvic cavity of the male, the bladder is located immediately behind the pubic bones and in front of the rectum on the median sagittal plane. The typical relationship of these structures is seen best in the CT. In Plate 5-5 on each side of the midline, the ampulla of the vas deferens and portions of the vesical venous plexus can be seen on the posterior wall of the bladder. In Plate 5-6, the plane of the section is slightly lower and a seminal vesicle can be seen on each side on the posterior wall of the bladder just lateral to the vas deferens. Anteriorly, in Plates 5-5 and 5-6 the inferior border of the anterior abdominal wall, just above the pubic symphysis, is included in the sections. The lower fibers of the internal abdominal oblique and rectus abdominis muscle are seen in Plate 5-5. Notice that the

ischial spine is included in the section in Plates 5-5 and 5-5 CT. A notch indicating the medial portion of the obturator canal is identified in Plate 5-6 and can also be seen in Plate 5-5 CT. The coccygeus muscle, which forms the posterior portion of the pelvic diaphragm, is identified in Plates 5-5 and 5-6.

In all three plates, muscles, vessels, and nerves of the upper thigh and gluteal region can be seen. Many of the muscles included in these plates have attachment to one or more of the bones of the pelvis. In Plate 5-6 on each side of the pelvis, the plane of section includes the tendon of the obturator internus muscle as it crosses the lesser sciatic notch of the ischium. The hip joint can be seen in each of these plates. In Plate 5-5, the ligament of the head of the femur is clearly visible on both sides. In Plate 5-6, the cavity and fibrous capsule of the hip joint are best studied on the left side. In examining the femur and studying the relationships of the muscles to it, notice that the sections shown in Plates 5-5 CT and 5-6 pass at approximately the same level through the head and greater trochanter of the femur. The relationships of the gluteus maximus, medius, and minimus muscles are well illustrated in Plates 5-5 and 5-6. Also note that the femoral, obturator, and sciatic nerves are identified in Plates 5-5 and 5-6. These relatively large nerves are more difficult to see but can be identified in the CT.

Plate 5-5 CT
Transverse Section

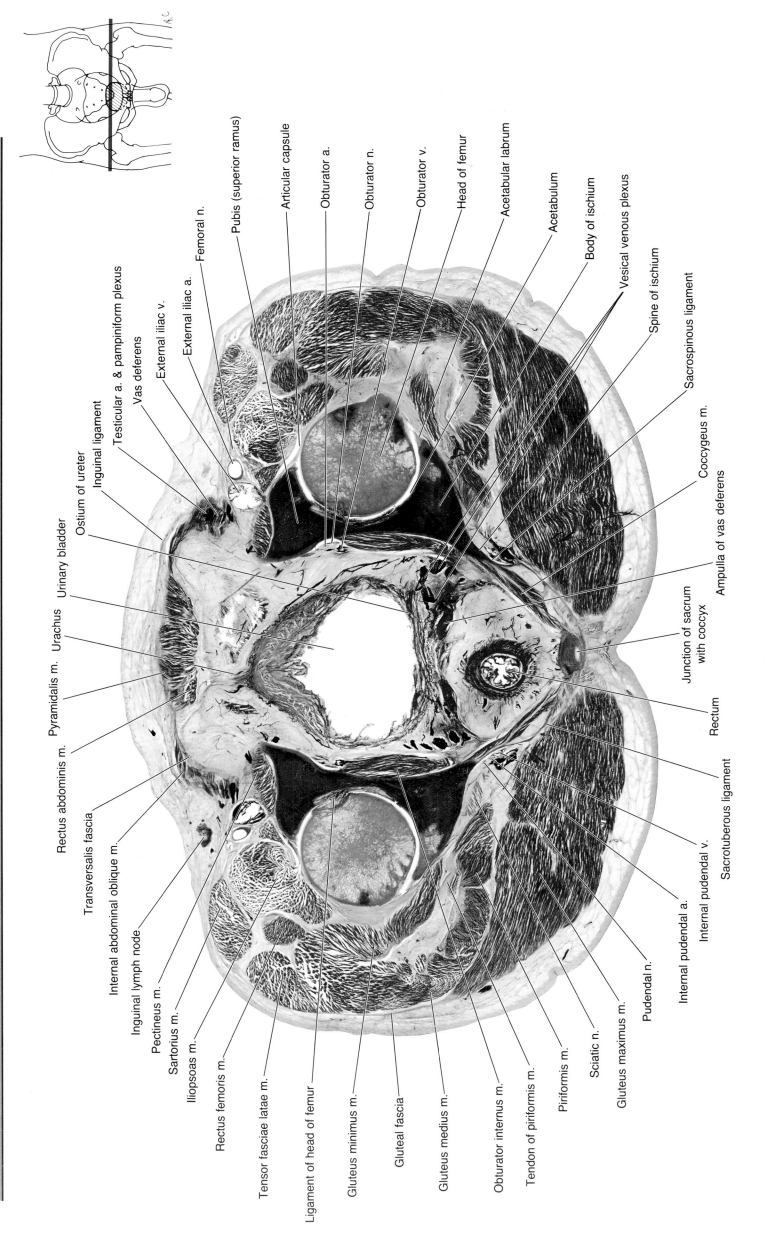

Pubis (superior ramus)

Articular capsule

Obturator a.

Obturator n.

Obturator v.

Head of femur

Acetabular labrum

Acetabulum

Body of ischium

Vesical venous plexus

Spine of ischium

Sacrospinous ligament

Coccygeus m.

Ampulla of vas deferens

Junction of sacrum with coccyx

Rectum

Sacrotuberous ligament

Internal pudendal a.

Internal pudendal v.

Pudendal n.

Sciatic n.

Gluteus maximus m.

Tendon of piriformis m.

Piriformis m.

Obturator internus m.

Gluteus medius m.

Gluteal fascia

Gluteus minimus m.

Ligament of head of femur

Tensor fasciae latae m.

Rectus femoris m.

Iliopsoas m.

Sartorius m.

Pectineus m.

Inguinal lymph node

Internal abdominal oblique m.

Transversalis fascia

Rectus abdominis m.   Pyramidalis m.   Urachus

Urinary bladder

Ostium of ureter

Inguinal ligament

Testicular a. & pampiniform plexus

Vas deferens

External iliac v.

External iliac a.

Femoral n.

MALE PELVIS AND
PERINEUM. Plate 5-5

Section through the pelvis passing approximately 7 cm below the anterosuperior iliac
spines and through the ischial spines. Bladder, rectum, and seminal vesicles are included.

Transverse Section

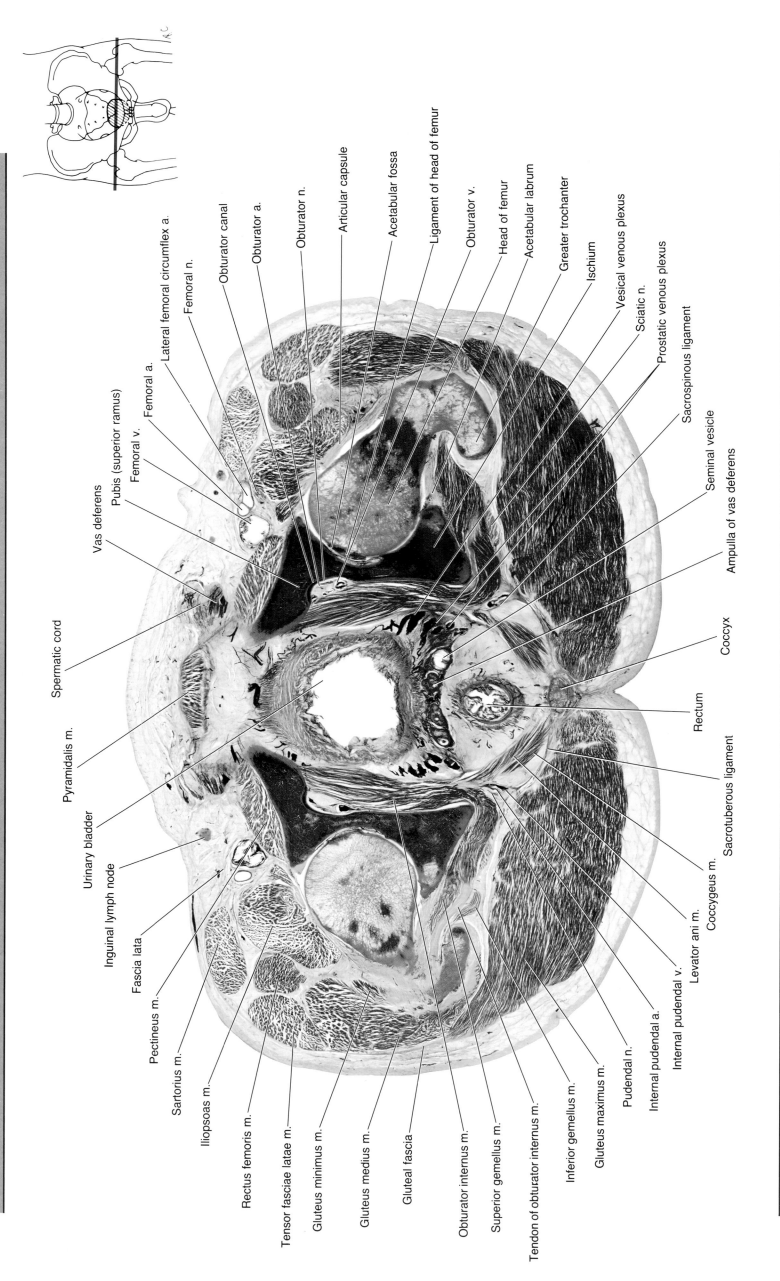

Obturator canal

Obturator a.

Obturator n.

Articular capsule

Acetabular fossa

Ligament of head of femur

Obturator v.

Head of femur

Acetabular labrum

Greater trochanter

Ischium

Vesical venous plexus

Sciatic n.

Prostatic venous plexus

Sacrospinous ligament

Seminal vesicle

Ampulla of vas deferens

Coccyx

Rectum

Sacrotuberous ligament

Coccygeus m.

Levator ani m.

Pudendal n.

Internal pudendal a.

Internal pudendal v.

Gluteus maximus m.

Inferior gemellus m.

Tendon of obturator internus m.

Superior gemellus m.

Obturator internus m.

Gluteal fascia

Gluteus medius m.

Gluteus minimus m.

Tensor fasciae latae m.

Rectus femoris m.

Iliopsoas m.

Sartorius m.

Pectineus m.

Inguinal lymph node

Fascia lata

Urinary bladder

Pyramidalis m.

Spermatic cord

Vas deferens

Pubis (superior ramus)

Femoral v.

Femoral a.

Femoral n.

Lateral femoral circumflex a.

MALE PELVIS AND
PERINEUM.   Plate 5-6

Section through the pelvis passing approximately 8 cm below the anterosuperior iliac
spines and the greater trochanter of each femur. Bladder and seminar vesicles are included.

Transverse Section

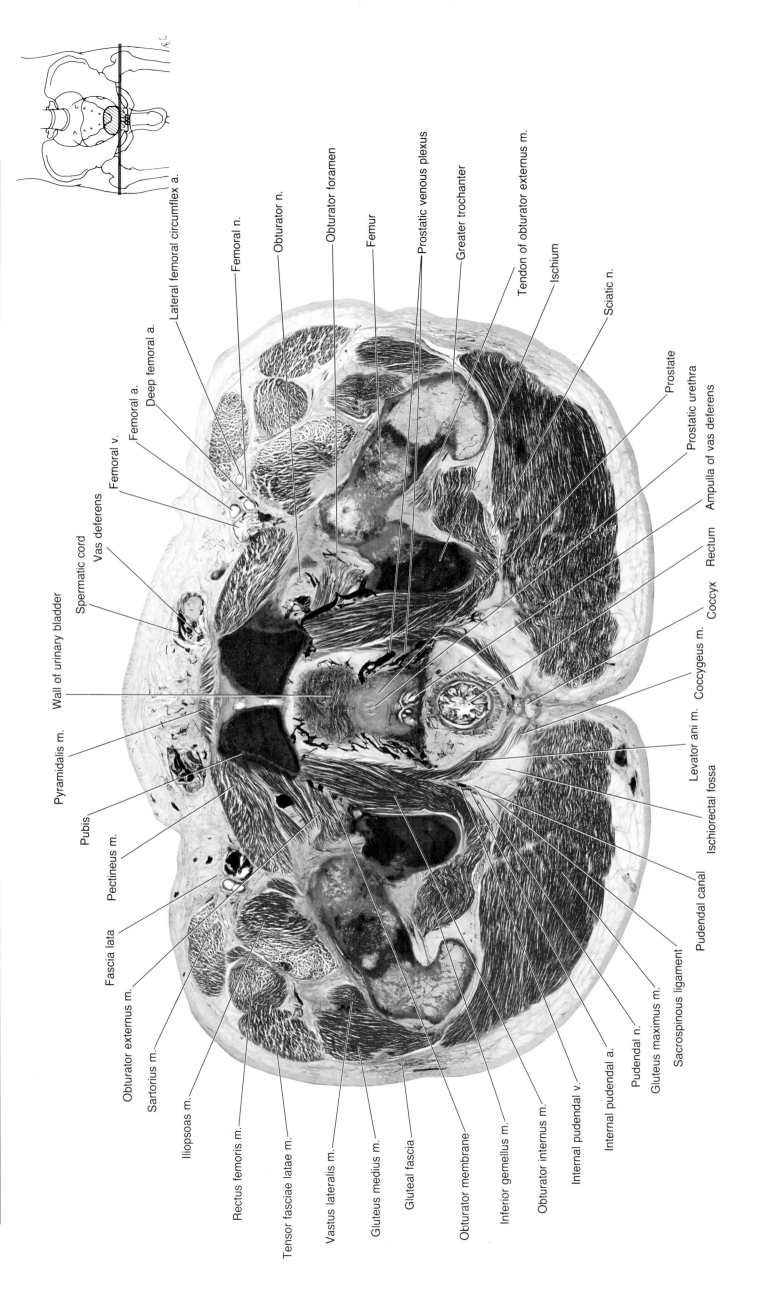

Lateral femoral circumflex a.

Femoral n.

Obturator n.

Obturator foramen

Femur

Prostatic venous plexus

Greater trochanter

Tendon of obturator externus m.

Ischium

Sciatic n.

Deep femoral a.

Femoral a.

Femoral v.

Vas deferens

Spermatic cord

Wall of urinary bladder

Pyramidalis m.

Pubis

Pectineus m.

Fascia lata

Obturator externus m.

Sartorius m.

Iliopsoas m.

Rectus femoris m.

Tensor fasciae latae m.

Vastus lateralis m.

Gluteus medius m.

Gluteal fascia

Obturator membrane

Inferior gemellus m.

Obturator internus m.

Internal pudendal v.

Internal pudendal a.

Pudendal n.

Gluteus maximus m.

Sacrospinous ligament

Pudendal canal

Ischiorectal fossa

Levator ani m.

Coccygeus m.

Coccyx

Rectum

Ampulla of vas deferens

Prostatic urethra

Prostate

MALE PELVIS AND
PERINEUM.   Plate 5-7

Section through the pelvis passing approximately 9 cm below the anterosuperior iliac
spines and the greater trochanter of each femur. Prostate and base of bladder are included.

Transverse Section

Spermatic cord

Femoral vessels

Inferior ramus of pubis

Prostate

Femur

Levator ani m.

Tuberosity of ischium

Rectum

Ischiorectal fossa

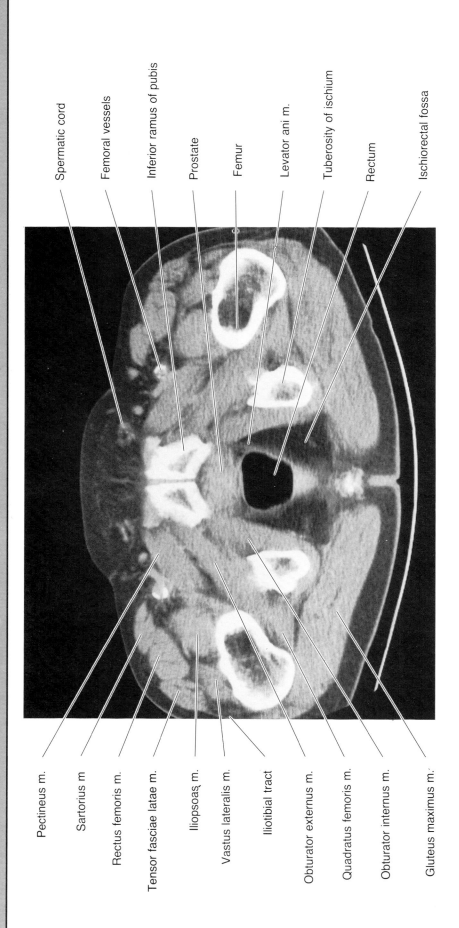

Pectineus m.

Sartorius m

Rectus femoris m.

Tensor fasciae latae m.

Iliopsoas m.

Vastus lateralis m.

Iliotibial tract

Obturator externus m.

Quadratus femoris m.

Obturator internus m.

Gluteus maximus m.

The sections shown in Plate 5-8 and the accompanying CT (Plate 5-8 CT) pass in transverse planes through the pelvis at the level of the obturator foramen and through the neck and greater trochanter of the femur.

As was explained in the legend of Plate 5-5, the pelvic diaphragm divides the cavity of the true pelvis into the main pelvic cavity above the muscle layer and the perineum below. In Plate 5-8 and 5-8 CT, the sections pass through the main pelvic cavity inferior to the bladder and include the prostate and rectum. In Plate 5-8, the prostatic urethra is identified as it passes through the prostate. The prostatic venous plexus that surrounds the prostate also can be seen. Adjacent to the rectum, a portion of the coccygeus muscle, which forms the posterior portion of the pelvic diaphragm, is identified in both plates. The ischiorectal fossa lies further lateral to rectum and is bounded medially by the pelvic diaphragm, laterally by the ischial tuberosity and fascia of the obturator internus muscle,

and posteriorly by the lower border of the gluteus maximus muscle. In Plate 5-8, the pudendal nerve and internal pudendal artery and vein are identified on the lateral wall of the ischiorectal fossa within the pudendal(Alcock's) canal formed by the lower part of the obturator internus fascia. The spermatic cord is identified in both plates anterolateral to the pubic symphysis.

In both plates, muscles, vessels, and nerves of the upper thigh and gluteal region can be seen. All of the muscles included in these two plates have an attachment to one or more of the bones of the pelvis. On both sides of Plate 5-8, the orientation of the Obturator internus and externus muscles are well defined as they attach to the obturator membrane and the inner and outer aspects, respectively, of the bones forming the obturator foramen. The femoral, obturator, and sciatic nerves are identified in Plate 5-8. These relatively large nerves are more difficult to identify in the CT.

Plate 5-8 CT
Transverse Section

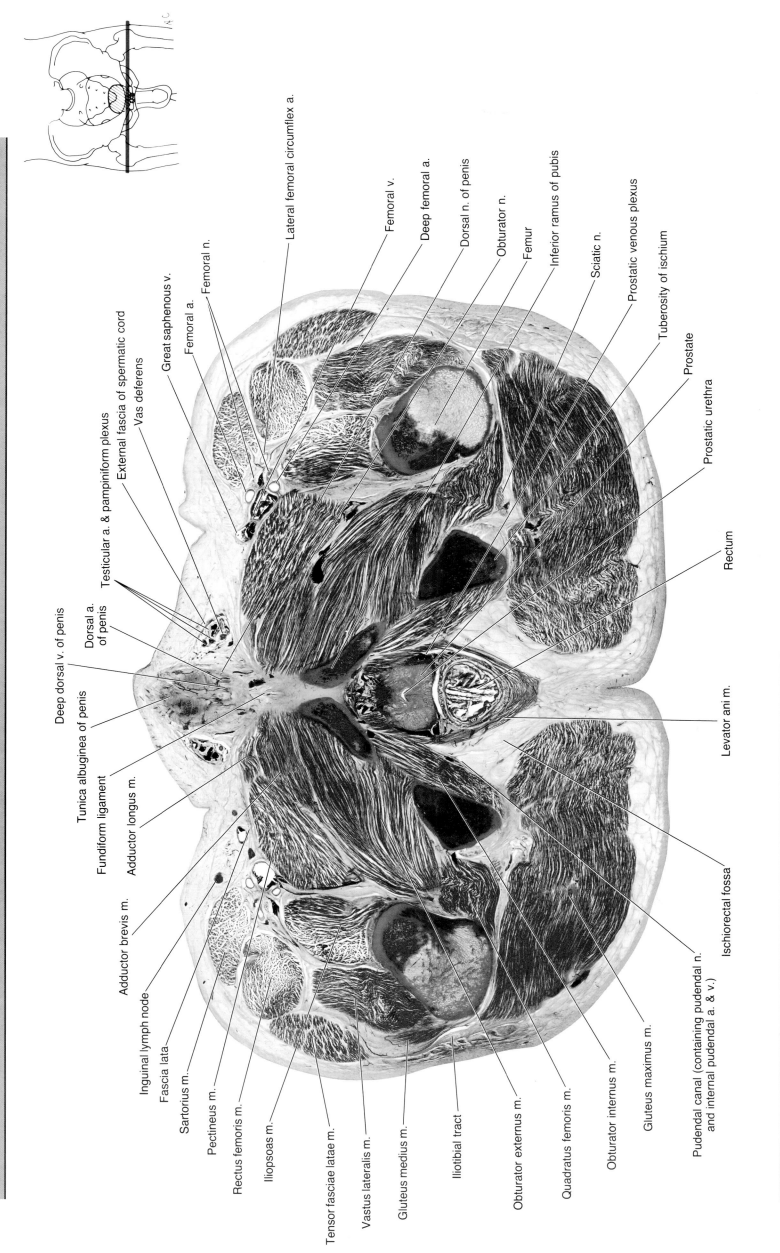

Lateral femoral circumflex a.

Femoral v.

Deep femoral a.

Dorsal n. of penis

Obturator n.

Femur

Inferior ramus of pubis

Sciatic n.

Prostatic venous plexus

Tuberosity of ischium

Prostate

Prostatic urethra

Femoral n.

Femoral a.

Great saphenous v.

Vas deferens

External fascia of spermatic cord

Testicular a. & pampiniform plexus

Dorsal a. of penis

Deep dorsal v. of penis

Tunica albuginea of penis

Fundiform ligament

Adductor longus m.

Adductor brevis m.

Inguinal lymph node

Fascia lata

Sartorius m.

Pectineus m.

Rectus femoris m.

Iliopsoas m.

Tensor fasciae latae m.

Vastus lateralis m.

Gluteus medius m.

Iliotibial tract

Obturator externus m.

Quadratus femoris m.

Obturator internus m.

Gluteus maximus m.

Pudendal canal (containing pudendal n. and internal pudendal a. & v.)

Ischiorectal fossa

Rectum

Levator ani m.

MALE PELVIS AND
PERINEUM.   Plate 5-8

Section through the pelvis passing approximately 11 cm below the anterosuperior iliac
spines and the neck of the right femur. Prostate, rectum, and dorsum of penis are included.

Transverse Section

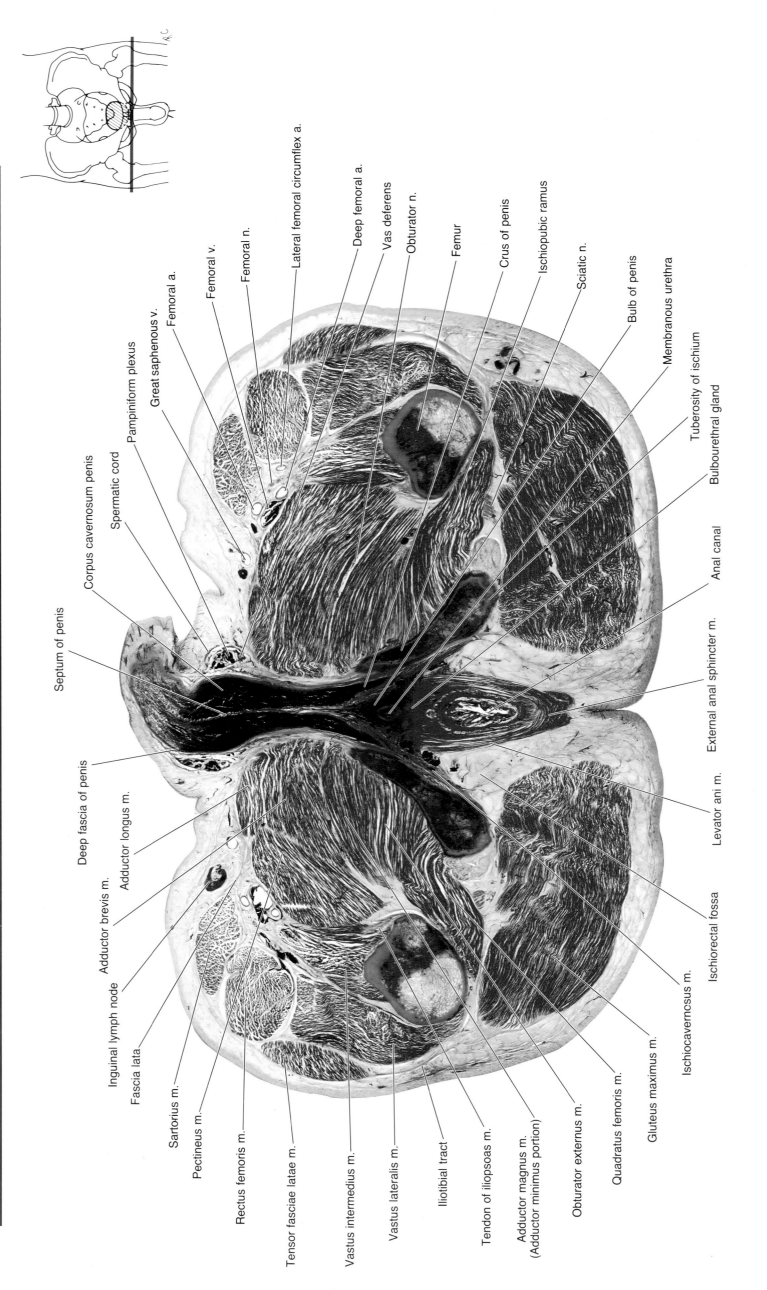

Septum of penis

Deep fascia of penis

Inguinal lymph node

Fascia lata

Sartorius m.

Pectineus m.

Rectus femoris m.

Tensor fasciae latae m.

Vastus intermedius m.

Vastus lateralis m.

Iliotibial tract

Tendon of iliopsoas m.

Adductor magnus m. (Adductor minimus portion)

Obturator externus m.

Quadratus femoris m.

Gluteus maximus m.

Ischiocaverncsus m.

Ischiorectal fossa

Levator ani m.

External anal sphincter m.

Anal canal

Bulbourethral gland

Tuberosity of ischium

Membranous urethra

Bulb of penis

Sciatic n.

Ischiopubic ramus

Crus of penis

Femur

Obturator n.

Vas deferens

Deep femoral a.

Lateral femoral circumflex a.

Femoral n.

Femoral v.

Femoral a.

Great saphenous v.

Pampiniform plexus

Spermatic cord

Corpus cavernosum penis

Adductor longus m.

Adductor brevis m.

MALE PELVIS AND
PERINEUM. Plate 5-9

Section through the pelvis passing approximately 12 cm below the anterosuperior iliac
spines and the lesser trochanter of each femur. Rectum and root of the penis are included.

Transverse Section

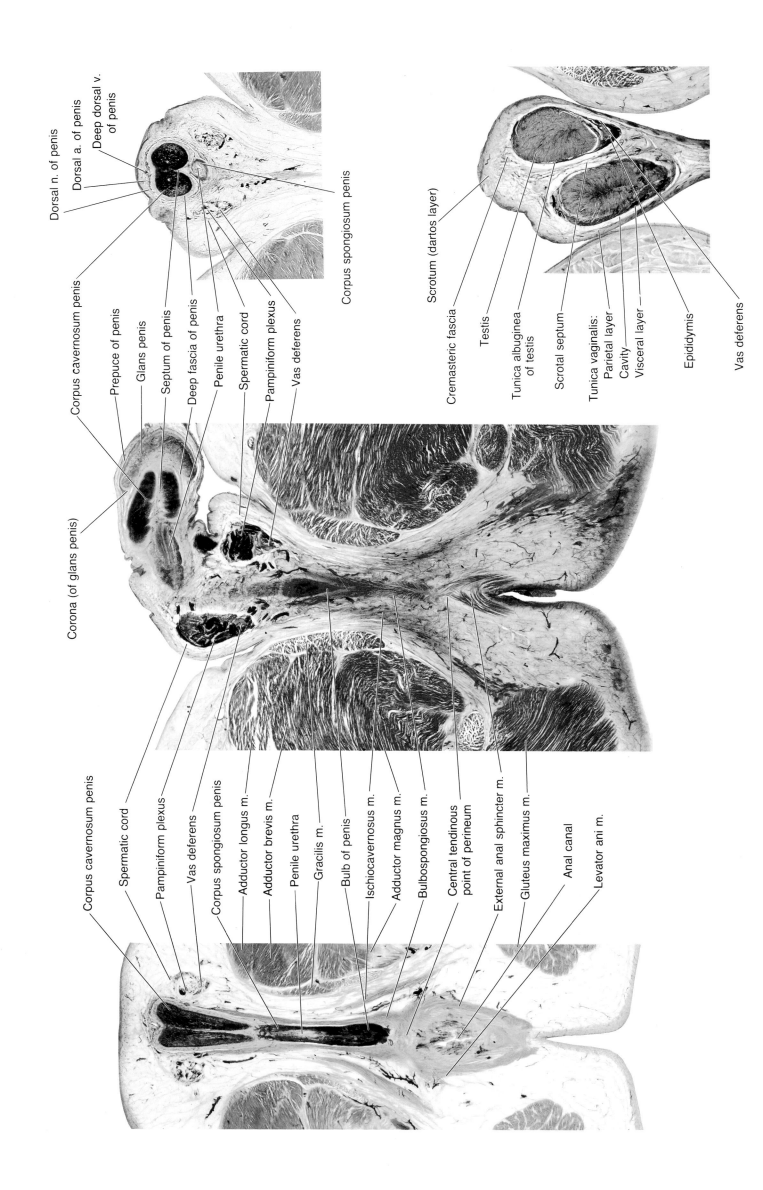

Dorsal n. of penis
Dorsal a. of penis
Deep dorsal v. of penis
Corpus spongiosum penis

Corpus cavernosum penis
Prepuce of penis
Glans penis
Septum of penis
Deep fascia of penis
Penile urethra
Spermatic cord
Pampiniform plexus
Vas deferens

Corona (of glans penis)

Corpus cavernosum penis
Spermatic cord
Pampiniform plexus
Vas deferens
Corpus spongiosum penis
Adductor longus m.
Adductor brevis m.
Penile urethra
Gracilis m.
Bulb of penis
Ischiocavernosus m.
Adductor magnus m.
Bulbospongiosus m.
Central tendinous point of perineum
External anal sphincter m.
Gluteus maximus m.
Anal canal
Levator ani m.

Scrotum (dartos layer)
Cremasteric fascia
Testis
Tunica albuginea of testis
Scrotal septum
Tunica vaginalis:
Parietal layer
Cavity
Visceral layer
Epididymis
Vas deferens

MALE PELVIS AND
PERINEUM. Plates 5-10 through 5-13

Series of transverse sections through the root of the penis and scrotum.

Part VI

Female Pelvis and
Perineum

Plates 6-1 to 6-6

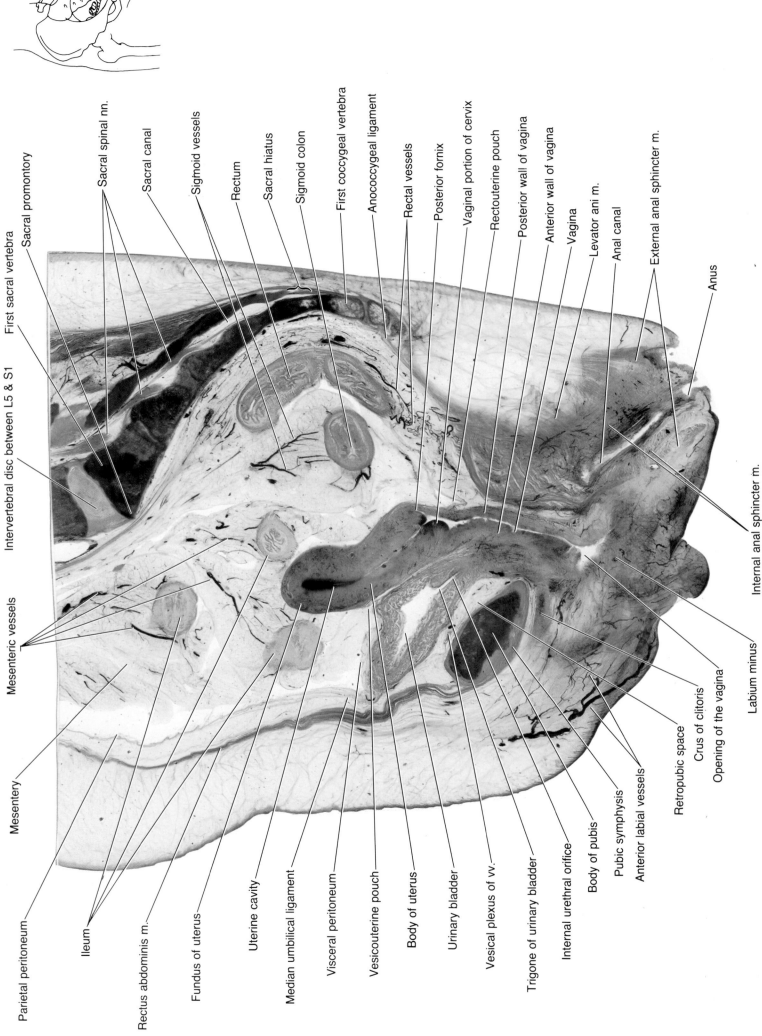

Parietal peritoneum

Mesentery

Mesenteric vessels

Intervertebral disc between L5 & S1

First sacral vertebra

Sacral promontory

Sacral spinal nn.

Sacral canal

Sigmoid vessels

Rectum

Sacral hiatus

Sigmoid colon

First coccygeal vertebra

Anococcygeal ligament

Rectal vessels

Posterior fornix

Vaginal portion of cervix

Rectouterine pouch

Posterior wall of vagina

Anterior wall of vagina

Vagina

Levator ani m.

Anal canal

External anal sphincter m.

Anus

Ileum

Rectus abdominis m.

Fundus of uterus

Uterine cavity

Median umbilical ligament

Visceral peritoneum

Vesicouterine pouch

Body of uterus

Urinary bladder

Vesical plexus of vv.

Trigone of urinary bladder

Internal urethral orifice

Body of pubis

Pubic symphysis

Anterior labial vessels

Retropubic space

Crus of clitoris

Opening of the vagina

Labium minus

Internal anal sphincter m.

FEMALE PELVIS AND
PERINEUM.   Plate 6-1

Sagittal Section

The plane of section passes slightly to the left of the median plane. The vesicouterine and rectouterine pouches and
bladder, vagina, and rectum are included in the section. The uterus is in an anteverted and retroflexed position.

Aponeurosis of external abdominal oblique m.

Internal abdominal oblique m.

External iliac a.

External iliac

Left ureter

Internal pudendal v.

Internal pudendal a.

Internal iliac v.

Superior gluteal n.

Superior gluteal vessels

Sacral plexus

Inferior gluteal a.

Oviduct

Rectum

Sacral canal

Fourth sacral vertebra

Uterine cavity

Uterus

Piriformis m.

Right ureter

Ovary

Gluteus maximus m.

Gluteus medius m.

Gluteus minimus m.

Gluteal fascia

Greater omentum

Femoral n.

Iliopsoas m.

Body of ilium

Sartorius m.

Tensor fasciae latae m.

Small intestine

Rectus abdominis m.

Mesentery

Sigmoid colon

FEMALE PELVIS AND
PERINEUM.   Plate 6-2

Section through the false pelvis passing approximately 4 cm below the anterosuperior iliac spines. The body of the uterus, ovaries and oviducts are included in the section. The uterus is enlarged and is in an abnormal posterior position.

Transverse Section

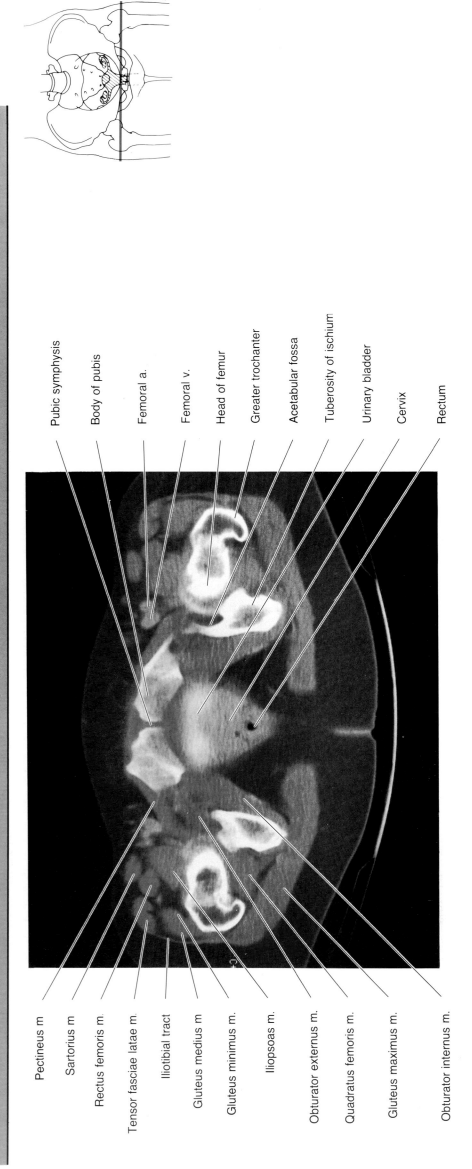

Pectineus m

Sartorius m

Rectus femoris m.

Tensor fasciae latae m.

Iliotibial tract

Gluteus medius m

Gluteus minimus m.

Iliopsoas m.

Obturator externus m.

Quadratus femoris m.

Gluteus maximus m.

Obturator internus m.

Pubic symphysis

Body of pubis

Femoral a.

Femoral v.

Head of femur

Greater trochanter

Acetabular fossa

Tuberosity of ischium

Urinary bladder

Cervix

Rectum

The sections shown in Plate 6-3 and the accompanying CT (Plate 6-3 CT) pass in transverse planes through the pelvis and femur. Note that in both plates the plane of the section is slightly oblique from left to right. On the right side, the section includes the head of the femur, greater trochanter, and the lower aspect of the acetabulum. The plane passes slightly lower on the left side. Therefore, the lower aspect of the greater trochanter is included as the plane of section passes through the femur.

The pelvic diaphragm, composed of the levator ani and coccygeus muscles, divides the cavity of the true pelvis into the main pelvic cavity above and the perineum below. In the main pelvic cavity of the female, the bladder, uterus and vagina, and rectum are located in the median sagittal plane from anterior to posterior in the order in which they are listed. As is also seen in the male, the urinary bladder is located immediately behind the pubic bones. In both plates the plane of section passes through the cervix and includes the upper portion of the vagina. However, this relationship is best seen in Plate 6-3. As seen in Plate 6-3, the rectum deviates further to the left of the median sagittal plane than is normal. This apparently is the result of enlargement and pathological changes in the uterus in the specimen shown. A more typical relationship of the rectum and cervix and vagina is seen in the CT. The ischiorectal fossa lies lateral to rectum and is bounded medially by the pelvic diaphragm, laterally by the ischial tuberosity and fascia of the obturator internus muscle, and posteriorly by the lower border of the gluteus maximus muscle. In Plate 6-3, the pudendal nerve and internal pudendal artery and vein are identified on the lateral wall of the ischiorectal fossa within the pudendal (Alcock's) canal formed by the lower part of the obturator internus fascia.

In both plates, muscles included in these two plates have an attachment to one or more of the bones seen. All of the muscles included in this section are well seen. On the right side of Plate 6-3, the orientation of the Obturator internus and externus muscles are well defined as they attach to the obturator membrane and the inner and outer aspects, respectively, of the bones forming the obturator foramen. On the left side, the plane of section is slightly higher and includes the tendon of the obturator internus muscle as it crosses the lesser sciatic notch of the ischium. The cavity and fibrous capsule of the hip joint also can be seen on the left side. The femoral, obturator, and sciatic nerves are identified in Plate 6-3. These relatively large nerves are more difficult to identify in the CT.

Plate 6-3 CT
Transverse Section

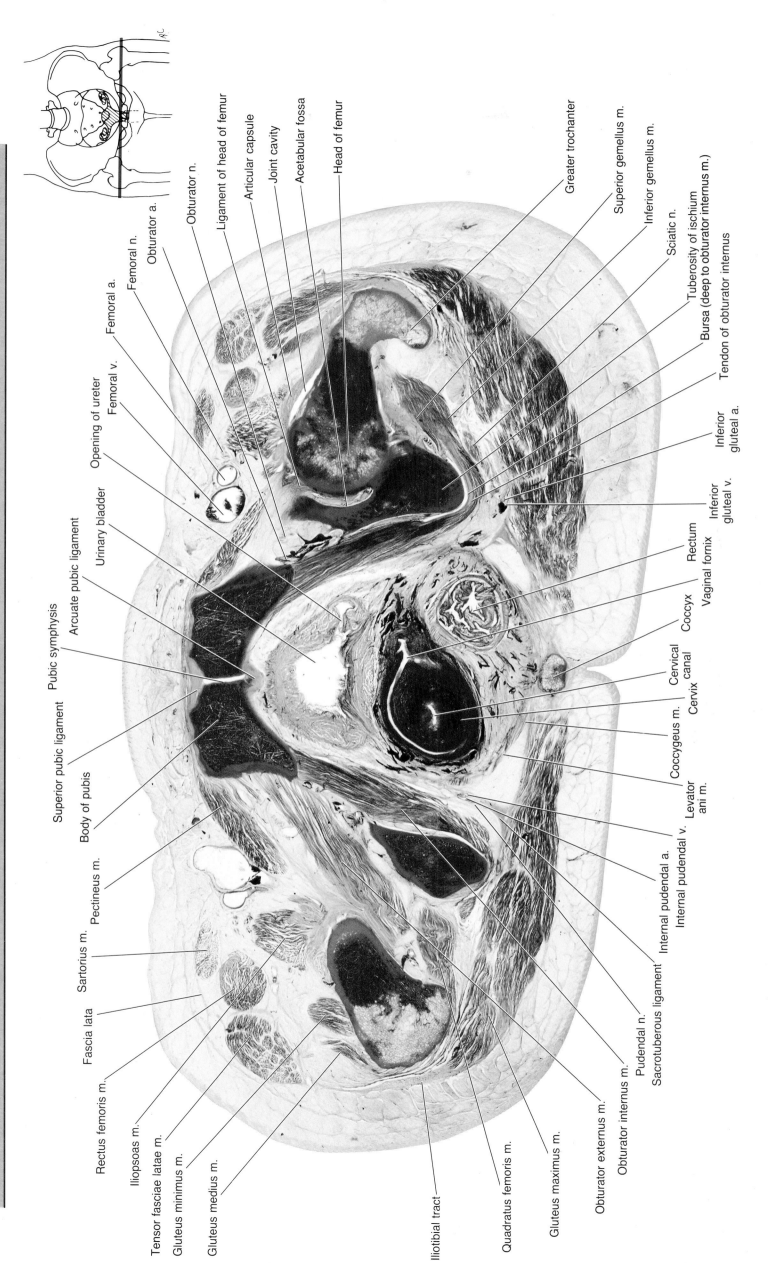

Rectus femoris m.

Fascia lata Sartorius m. Pectineus m.

Iliopsoas m.

Tensor fasciae latae m.

Gluteus minimus m.

Gluteus medius m.

Superior pubic ligament Pubic symphysis

Body of pubis Arcuate pubic ligament

Urinary bladder

Opening of ureter

Femoral v.

Femoral a.

Femoral n.

Obturator a.

Obturator n.

Ligament of head of femur

Articular capsule

Joint cavity

Acetabular fossa

Head of femur

Greater trochanter

Superior gemellus m.

Inferior gemellus m.

Sciatic n.

Tuberosity of ischium

Bursa (deep to obturator internus m.)

Tendon of obturator internus

Inferior gluteal a.

Inferior gluteal v.

Rectum

Vaginal fornix

Coccyx

Cervix Cervical canal

Coccygeus m.

Levator ani m.

Internal pudendal v.

Internal pudendal a.

Pudendal n.

Sacrotuberous ligament

Obturator internus m.

Obturator externus m.

Quadratus femoris m.

Gluteus maximus m.

Iliotibial tract

FEMALE PELVIS AND
PERINEUM. Plate 6-3

Slightly oblique section through the pelvis passing approximately 10 cm on the right and 8 cm on
the left below the anterosuperior iliac spines. Bladder, cervix, and vagina are included.

Transverse Section

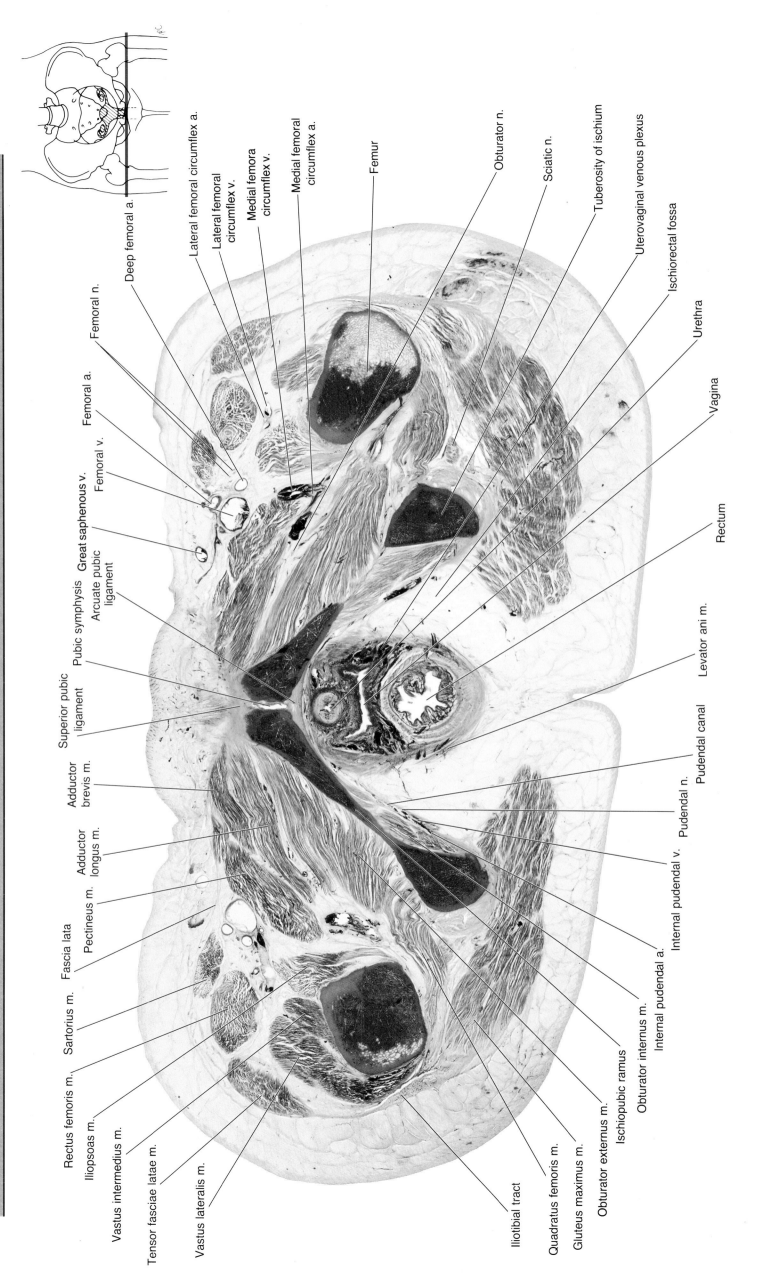

Deep femoral a.

Lateral femoral circumflex a.

Lateral femoral circumflex v.

Medial femoral circumflex v.

Medial femoral circumflex a.

Femur

Obturator n.

Sciatic n.

Tuberosity of ischium

Uterovaginal venous plexus

Ischiorectal fossa

Urethra

Vagina

Rectum

Levator ani m.

Pudendal canal

Pudendal n.

Internal pudendal v.

Internal pudendal a.

Obturator internus m.

Obturator externus m.

Ischiopubic ramus

Gluteus maximus m.

Quadratus femoris m.

Iliotibial tract

Femoral n.

Femoral a.

Femoral v.

Great saphenous v.

Pubic symphysis

Arcuate pubic ligament

Superior pubic ligament

Adductor brevis m.

Adductor longus m.

Pectineus m.

Fascia lata

Sartorius m.

Tensor fasciae latae m.

Vastus lateralis m.

Vastus intermedius m.

Iliopsoas m.

Rectus femoris m.

FEMALE PELVIS AND
PERINEUM.   Plate 6-4

Slightly oblique section through the pelvis passing approximately 12 cm on the right and 10 cm on
the left below the anterosuperior iliac spines. Urethra, vagina, and rectum are included.

Transverse Section

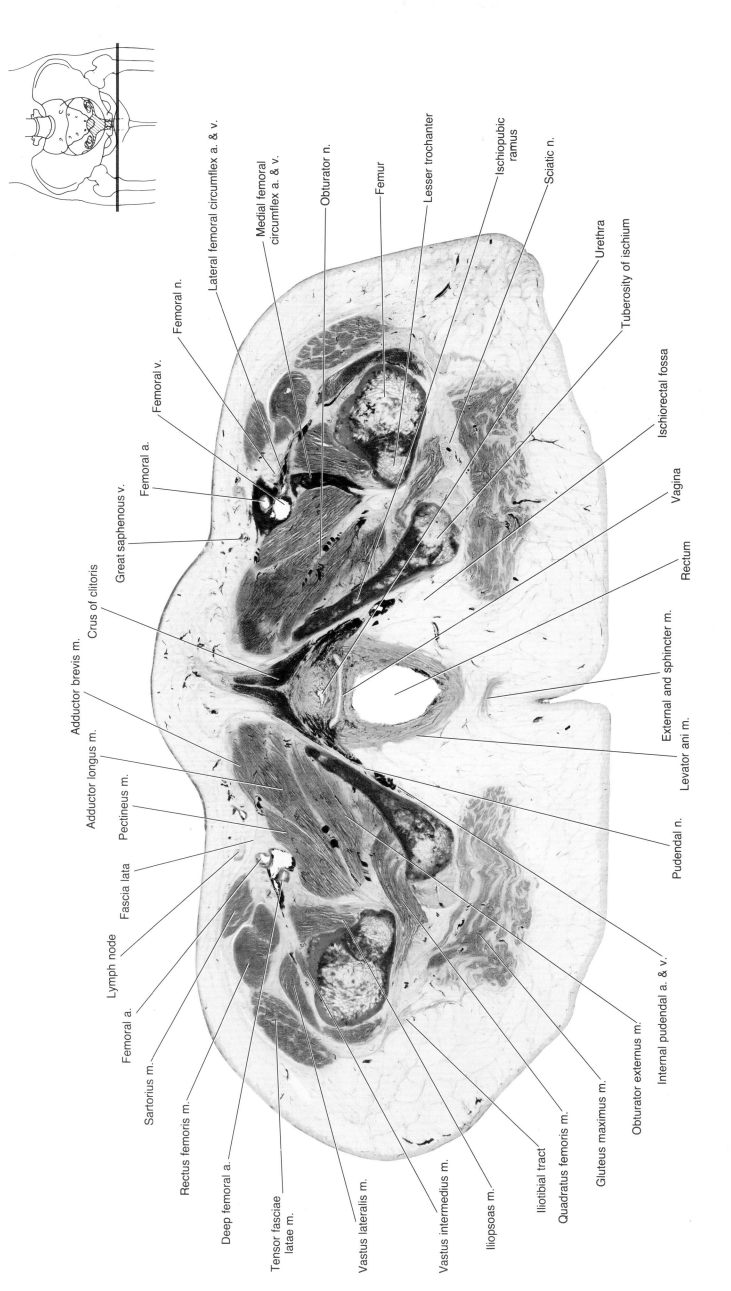

Lateral femoral circumflex a. & v.

Medial femoral circumflex a. & v.

Obturator n.

Femur

Lesser trochanter

Ischiopubic ramus

Sciatic n.

Urethra

Tuberosity of ischium

Ischiorectal fossa

Femoral n.

Femoral v.

Femoral a.

Great saphenous v.

Crus of clitoris

Adductor brevis m.

Adductor longus m.

Pectineus m.

Fascia lata

Lymph node

Femoral a.

Sartorius m.

Rectus femoris m.

Deep femoral a.

Tensor fasciae latae m.

Vastus lateralis m.

Vastus intermedius m.

Iliopsoas m.

Iliotibial tract

Quadratus femoris m.

Gluteus maximus m.

Obturator externus m.

Internal pudendal a. & v.

Pudendal n.

Levator ani m.

External and sphincter m.

Rectum

Vagina

FEMALE PELVIS AND
PERINEUM. Plate 6-5

Section passes through the lesser trochanter of the femur and through the pelvis approximately 13 cm below the anterosuperior iliac spines.
Urethra, vagina, and rectum are included.

Transverse Section

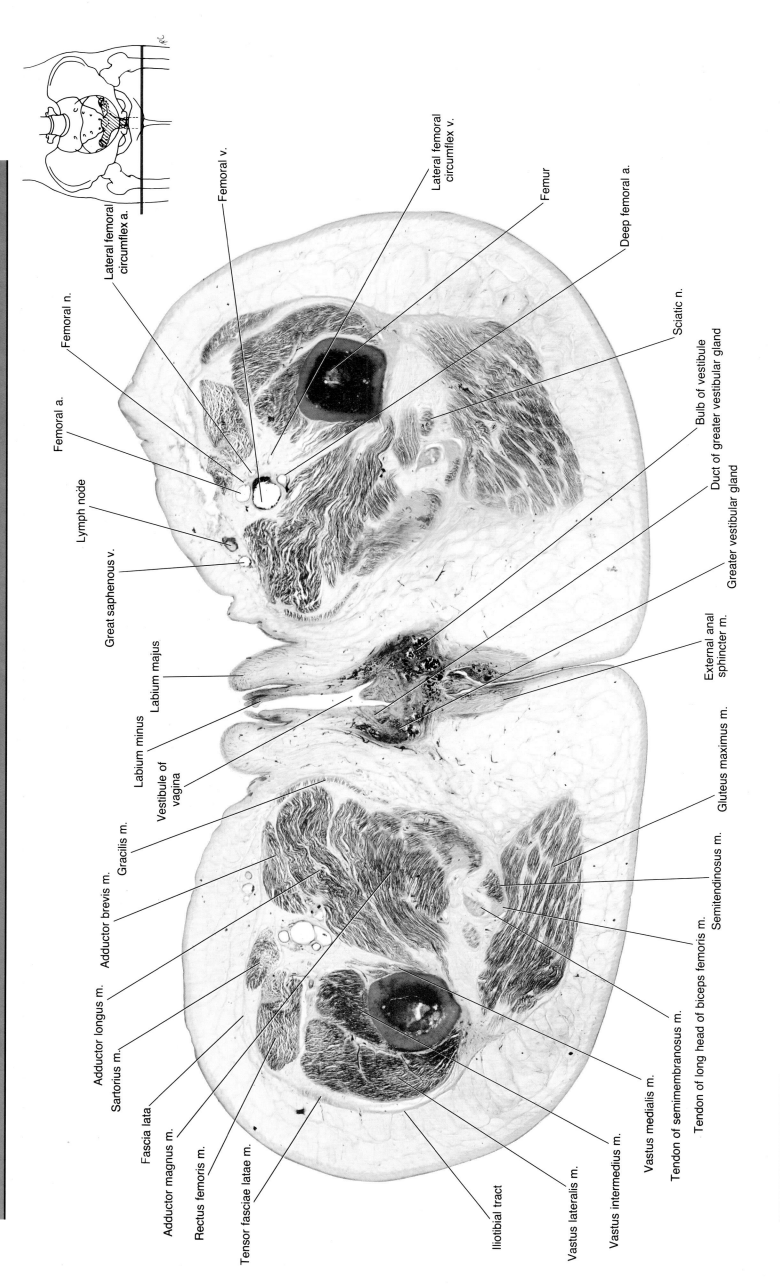

Lateral femoral
circumflex a.

Femoral n.

Femoral v.

Femoral a.

Lymph node

Great saphenous v.

Labium majus

Labium minus

Vestibule of
vagina

Gracilis m.

Adductor brevis m.

Adductor longus m.

Sartorius m.

Fascia lata

Adductor magnus m.

Rectus femoris m.

Tensor fasciae latae m.

Lateral femoral
circumflex v.

Femur

Deep femoral a.

Sciatic n.

Bulb of vestibule

Duct of greater vestibular gland

Greater vestibular gland

External anal
sphincter m.

Gluteus maximus m.

Semitendinosus m.

Tendon of semimembranosus m.

Tendon of long head of biceps femoris m.

Vastus medialis m.

Vastus lateralis m.

Vastus intermedius m.

Iliotibial tract

FEMALE PELVIS AND
PERINEUM.   Plate 6-6

Section passes through the pelvis approximately 15 cm below the anterosuperior iliac spines. Labia
majora and minor, vaginal vestibule, bulb of the vestibule and greater vestibular gland are included.

Transverse Section

Part VII

Lower Extremity

Plates 7-1 to 7-23

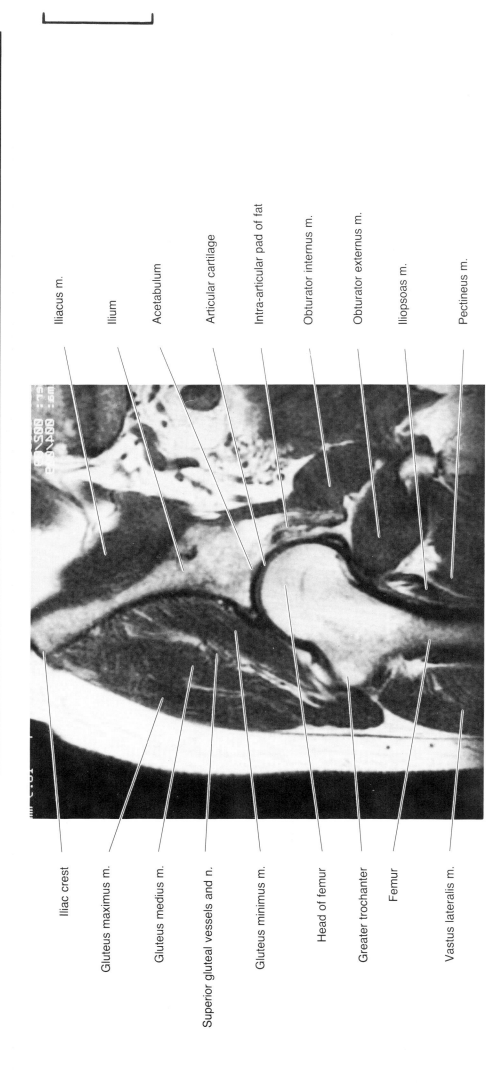

Iliacus m.

Ilium

Acetabulum

Articular cartilage

Intra-articular pad of fat

Obturator internus m.

Obturator externus m.

Iliopsoas m.

Pectineus m.

Iliac crest

Gluteus maximus m.

Gluteus medius m.

Superior gluteal vessels and n.

Gluteus minimus m.

Head of femur

Greater trochanter

Femur

Vastus lateralis m.

The sections shown in Plate 7-1 and the accompanying MRI (Plate 7-1 MRI) pass in a coronal plane through the head and greater trochanter of the femur and the hip joint. The head of the femur articulates with the cup-shaped acetabulum, which is deepened by the acetabular labrum. A fibrous capsule surrounds the femoral head as it extends from the acetabular margin to femur along the intertrochanteric line in front and along the posterior aspect of the neck of the femur behind. Externally the capsule is reinforced by three ligaments, namely the iliofemoral, pubofemoral, and ischiofemoral. The basic structure of the joint is well displayed in both Plates. However, the labrum, capsule, and portions of two of the extrinsic ligaments (the pubofemoral and ischiofemoral) can only be identified in Plate 7-1.

The capsule of the hip joint is surrounded by muscles. These include: anteriorly, the pectineus, iliopsoas, and rectus femoris muscles; superiorly, the piriformis and gluteus minimus muscles; posteriorly, the gemelli and quadratus femoris muscles and the tendon of obturator internus muscle; and, inferiorly, the obturator externus muscle. Several of these muscles can be identified in Plates 7-1 and 7-1 MRI. The obturator internus, externus, iliopsoas, and pectineus muscles are identified in both Plates. In Plate 7-1, the medial femoral circumflex artery and vein are identified as they pass between the iliopsoas and pectineus muscles. Above the hip joint the gluteus maximus, medius, and minimus muscles can be seen in both Plates. The superior gluteal vessels and nerve are identified as they pass in the plane between the gluteus medius and minimus muscles.

Plate 7-1 MRI
Coronal Section

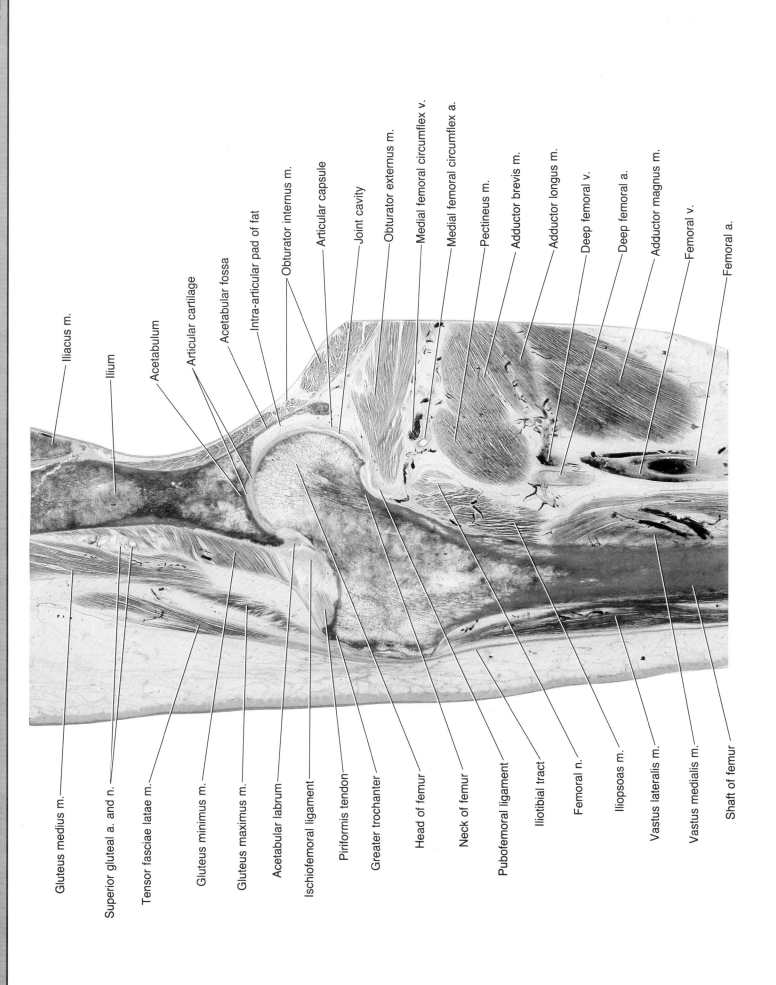

Gluteus medius m.

Superior gluteal a. and n.

Tensor fasciae latae m.

Gluteus minimus m.

Gluteus maximus m.

Acetabular labrum

Ischiofemoral ligament

Piriformis tendon

Greater trochanter

Head of femur

Neck of femur

Pubofemoral ligament

Iliotibial tract

Femoral n.

Iliopsoas m.

Vastus lateralis m.

Vastus medialis m.

Shaft of femur

Iliacus m.

Ilium

Acetabulum

Articular cartilage

Acetabular fossa

Intra-articular pad of fat

Obturator internus m.

Articular capsule

Joint cavity

Obturator externus m.

Medial femoral circumflex v.

Medial femoral circumflex a.

Pectineus m.

Adductor brevis m.

Adductor longus m.

Deep femoral v.

Deep femoral a.

Adductor magnus m.

Femoral v.

Femoral a.

LOWER EXTREMITY.
Plate 7-1

Section of the hip through the head of the femur and greater trochanter. The acetabulum and portions of
the ischiofemoral and pubofemoral ligaments are included.

Coronal Section

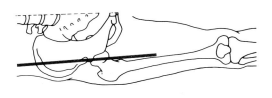

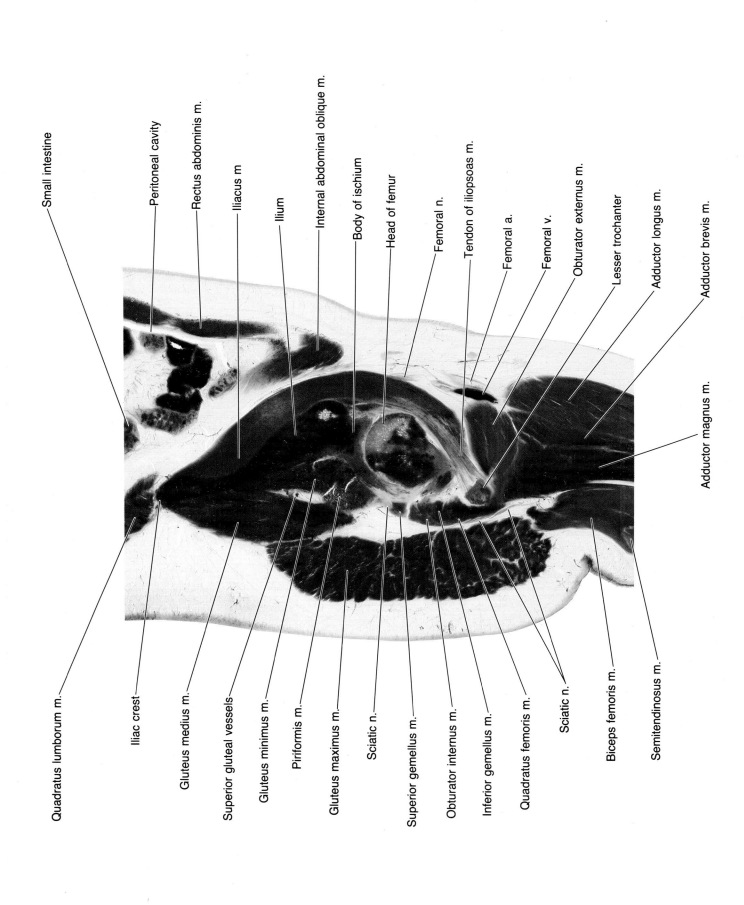

Quadratus lumborum m.

Iliac crest

Gluteus medius m.

Superior gluteal vessels

Gluteus minimus m.

Piriformis m.

Gluteus maximus m.

Sciatic n.

Superior gemellus m.

Obturator internus m.

Inferior gemellus m.

Quadratus femoris m.

Sciatic n.

Biceps femoris m.

Semitendinosus m.

Small intestine

Peritoneal cavity

Rectus abdominis m.

Iliacus m

Ilium

Internal abdominal oblique m.

Body of ischium

Head of femur

Femoral n.

Tendon of iliopsoas m.

Femoral a.

Femoral v.

Obturator externus m.

Lesser trochanter

Adductor longus m.

Adductor brevis m.

Adductor magnus m.

LOWER EXTREMITY.
Plate 7-2

Sagittal Section

Section of the hip through the medial aspect of the femoral head. The section includes the tendon of the iliopsoas muscle, the lesser trochanter, and Gluteus maximus, medius and minimus muscles.

Transverse Section

Superficial inguinal lymph node

Great saphenous v.

Adductor longus m.

Obturator n. - anterior division

Deep femoral v.

Deep femoral a.

Adductor brevis m.

Gracilis m.

Obturator n. - posterior division

Adductor magnus m.

Semimembranosus m.

Semitendinosus m.

Long head of biceps femoris m.

Sartorius m.

Femoral a.

Femoral n.

Femoral v.

Fascia lata

Rectus femoris m.

Tensor fasciae latae m.

Vastus intermedius m.

Vastus medialis m.

Vastus lateralis m.

Iliotibial tract

Shaft of femur

Iliopsoas m.

Lesser trochanter

Pectineus m.

Sciatic n.

Posterior femoral cutaneous n.

Gluteus maximus m.

LOWER EXTREMITY.
Plate 7-3

Section of the thigh through the lesser trochanter. The femoral vein, artery, and nerve are located just proximal to the adductor canal. The deep femoral artery and vein are included.

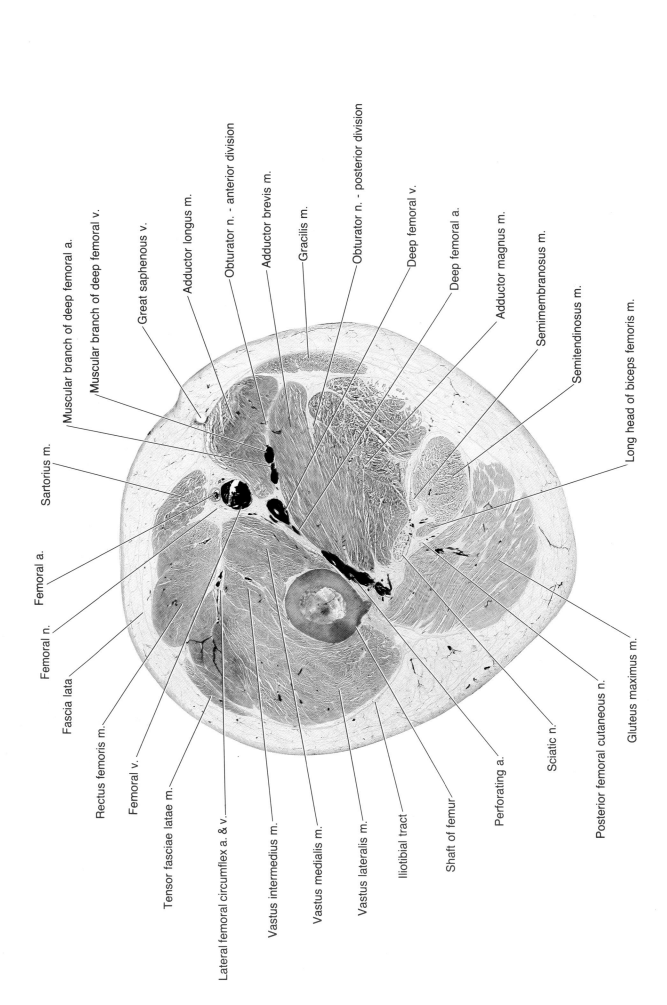

Sartorius m.

Femoral a.

Femoral n.

Fascia lata

Rectus femoris m.

Femoral v.

Tensor fasciae latae m.

Lateral femoral circumflex a. & v.

Vastus intermedius m.

Vastus medialis m.

Vastus lateralis m.

Iliotibial tract

Shaft of femur

Perforating a.

Sciatic n.

Posterior femoral cutaneous n.

Gluteus maximus m.

Muscular branch of deep femoral a.

Muscular branch of deep femoral v.

Great saphenous v.

Adductor longus m.

Obturator n. - anterior division

Adductor brevis m.

Gracilis m.

Obturator n. - posterior division

Deep femoral v.

Deep femoral a.

Adductor magnus m.

Semimembranosus m.

Semitendinosus m.

Long head of biceps femoris m.

Transverse Section

Section of the thigh through the proximal portion of the adductor canal. A perforating branch of the deep femoral artery is seen as it passes through the Adductor brevis.

LOWER EXTREMITY.
Plate 7-4

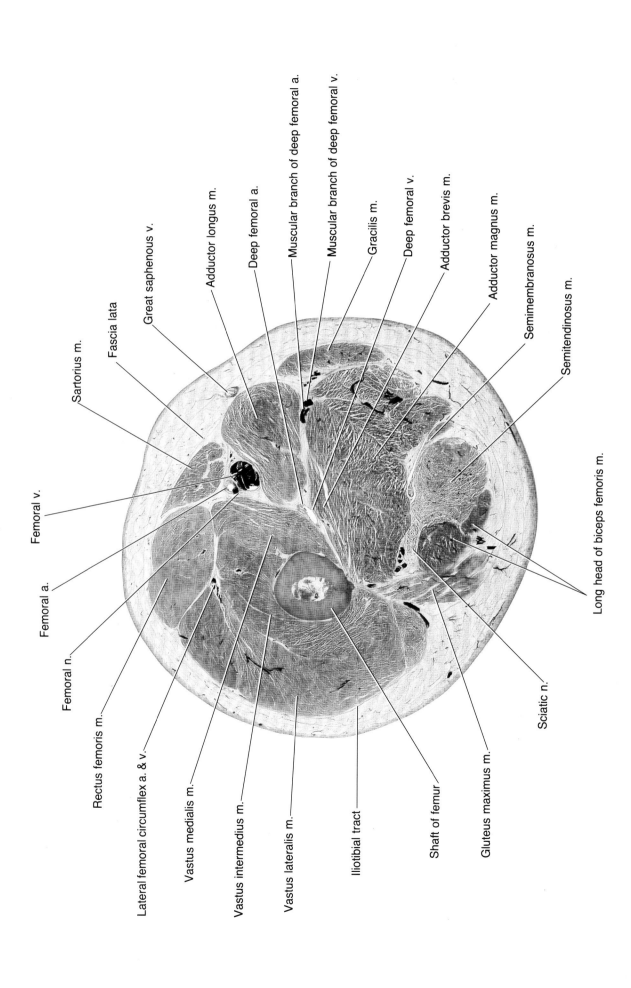

Femoral v.

Sartorius m.

Fascia lata

Great saphenous v.

Adductor longus m.

Deep femoral a.

Muscular branch of deep femoral a.

Muscular branch of deep femoral v.

Gracilis m.

Deep femoral v.

Adductor brevis m.

Adductor magnus m.

Semimembranosus m.

Semitendinosus m.

Long head of biceps femoris m.

Femoral a.

Femoral n.

Rectus femoris m.

Lateral femoral circumflex a. & v.

Vastus medialis m.

Vastus intermedius m.

Vastus lateralis m.

Iliotibial tract

Shaft of femur

Gluteus maximus m.

Sciatic n.

LOWER EXTREMITY.
Plate 7-5

Section of the thigh through the distal end of the attachment of the Gluteus maximus to the iliotibial tract, distal border of the Adductor brevis, and the adductor canal.

Transverse Section

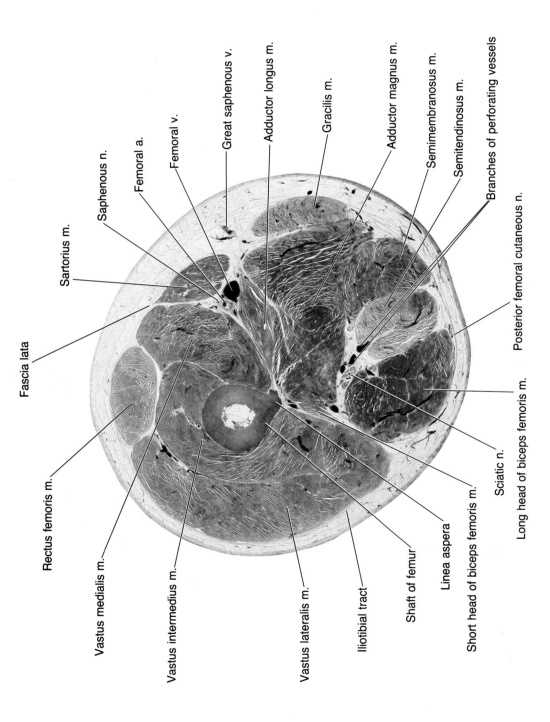

Fascia lata

Sartorius m.

Saphenous n.

Femoral a.

Femoral v.

Great saphenous v.

Adductor longus m.

Gracilis m.

Adductor magnus m.

Semimembranosus m.

Semitendinosus m.

Branches of perforating vessels

Posterior femoral cutaneous n.

Rectus femoris m.

Vastus medialis m.

Vastus intermedius m.

Vastus lateralis m.

Iliotibial tract

Shaft of femur

Linea aspera

Short head of biceps femoris m.

Sciatic n.

Long head of biceps femoris m.

LOWER EXTREMITY.
Plate 7-6

Section of the thigh through the distal end of the adductor canal.

Transverse Section

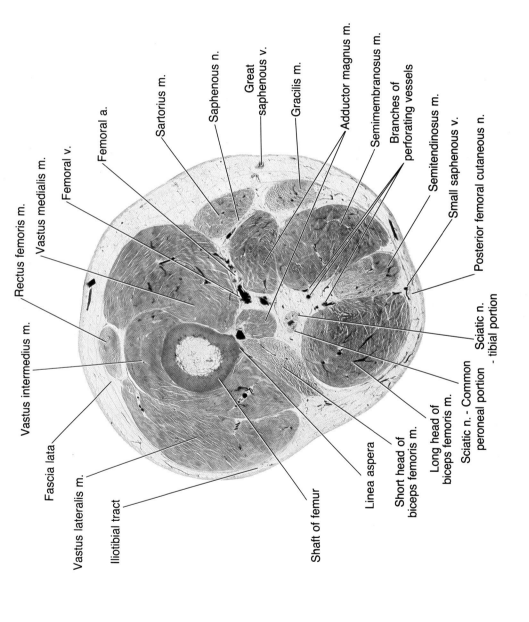

Vastus intermedius m.

Rectus femoris m.

Vastus medialis m.

Femoral v.

Femoral a.

Sartorius m.

Saphenous n.

Great
saphenous v.

Gracilis m.

Adductor magnus m.

Semimembranosus m.

Branches of
perforating vessels

Semitendinosus m.

Small saphenous v.

Posterior femoral cutaneous n.

Sciatic n.
- tibial portion

Sciatic n. - Common
peroneal portion

Long head of
biceps femoris m.

Short head of
biceps femoris m.

Linea aspera

Shaft of femur

Iliotibial tract

Vastus lateralis m.

Fascia lata

LOWER EXTREMITY.
Plate 7-7

Section of the thigh through the adductor hiatus.

Transverse Section

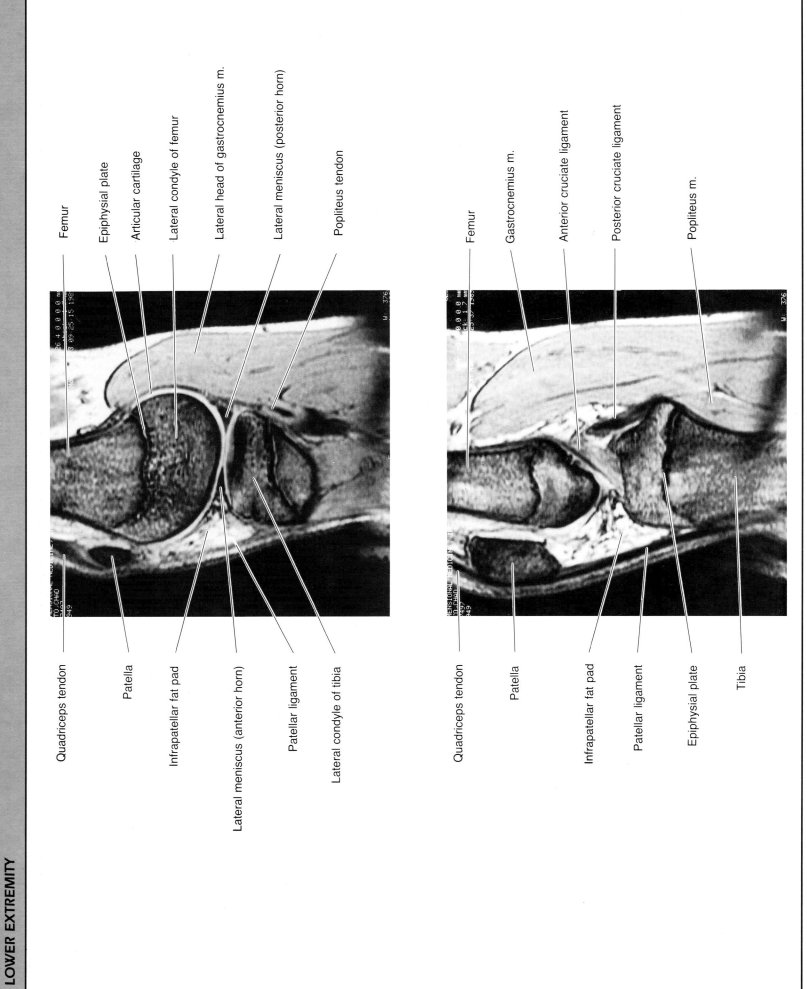

Quadriceps tendon

Patella

Infrapatellar fat pad

Lateral meniscus (anterior horn)

Patellar ligament

Lateral condyle of tibia

Femur

Epiphysial plate

Articular cartilage

Lateral condyle of femur

Lateral head of gastrocnemius m.

Lateral meniscus (posterior horn)

Popliteus tendon

Quadriceps tendon

Patella

Infrapatellar fat pad

Patellar ligament

Epiphysial plate

Tibia

Femur

Gastrocnemius m.

Anterior cruciate ligament

Posterior cruciate ligament

Popliteus m.

Plate 7-8 MRI
Sagittal Section

Plate 7-8 MRI: Section of the right knee passing through the lateral condyles of the femur and tibia.
Plate 7-9 MRI: Section of the right knee passing through the anterior and posterior cruciate ligaments.

Plate 7-9 MRI
Sagittal Section

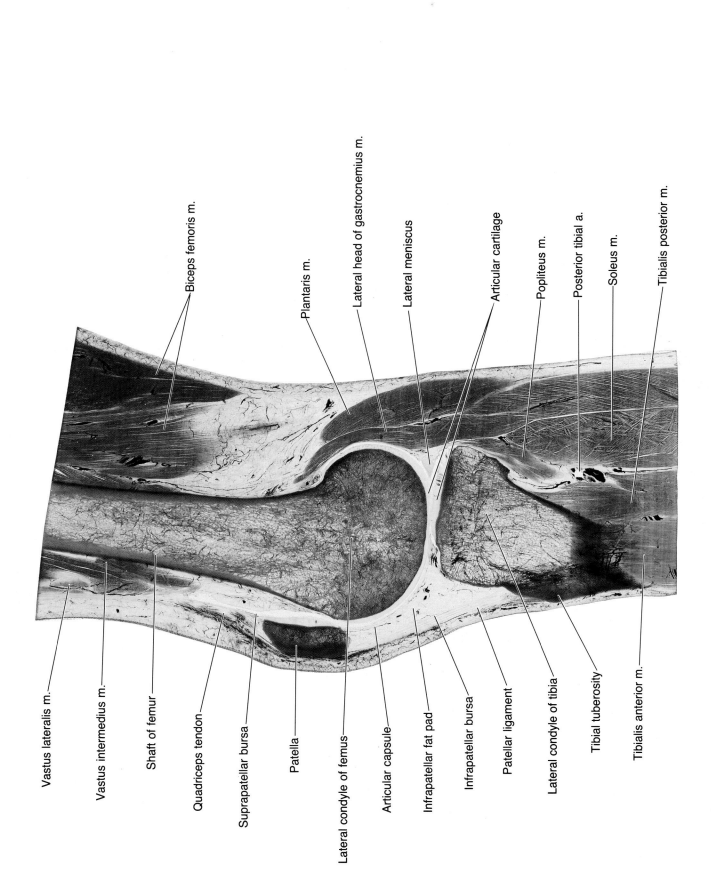

Vastus lateralis m.

Vastus intermedius m.

Shaft of femur

Quadriceps tendon

Suprapatellar bursa

Patella

Lateral condyle of femus

Articular capsule

Infrapatellar fat pad

Infrapatellar bursa

Patellar ligament

Lateral condyle of tibia

Tibial tuberosity

Tibialis anterior m.

Biceps femoris m.

Plantaris m.

Lateral head of gastrocnemius m.

Lateral meniscus

Articular cartilage

Popliteus m.

Posterior tibial a.

Soleus m.

Tibialis posterior m.

LOWER EXTREMITY.
Plate 7-8

Section of the right knee passing slightly lateral to the median plane and through the lateral condyles of the femur and tibia. Portions of the lateral meniscus can be identified in the section.

Sagittal Section

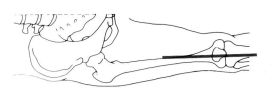

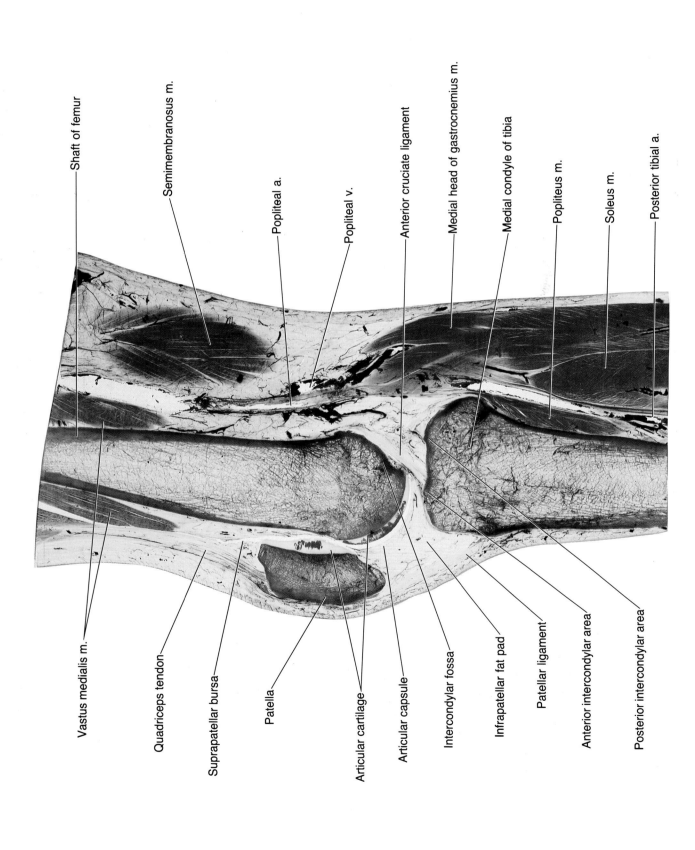

Shaft of femur

Semimembranosus m.

Popliteal a.

Popliteal v.

Anterior cruciate ligament

Medial head of gastrocnemius m.

Medial condyle of tibia

Popliteus m.

Soleus m.

Posterior tibial a.

Vastus medialis m.

Quadriceps tendon

Suprapatellar bursa

Patella

Articular cartilage

Articular capsule

Intercondylar fossa

Infrapatellar fat pad

Patellar ligament

Anterior intercondylar area

Posterior intercondylar area

LOWER EXTREMITY.
Plate 7-9

Section of the right knee passing through the anterior cruciate ligament and the intercondylar fossa of the
tibia. Portions of the popliteal vessels and tibial nerve are included in the section.

Sagittal Section

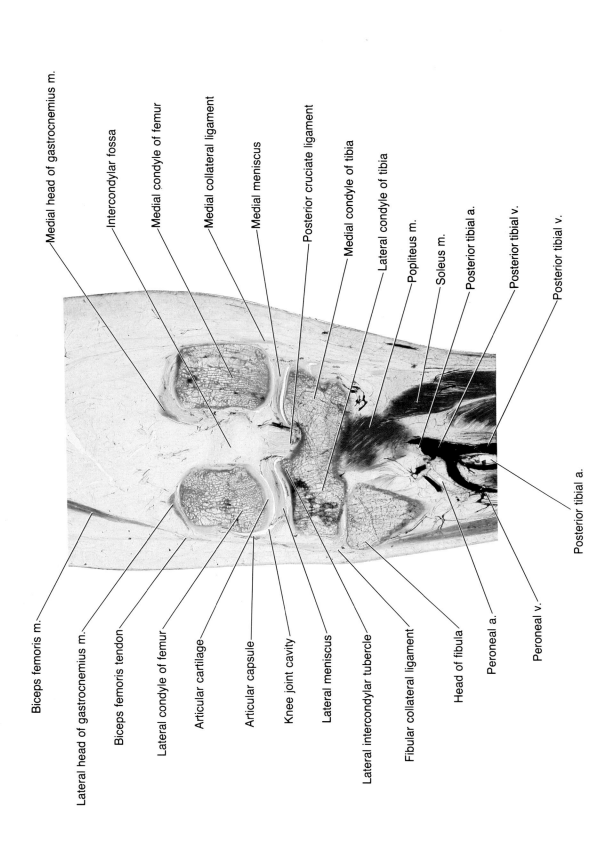

Medial head of gastrocnemius m.

Intercondylar fossa

Medial condyle of femur

Medial collateral ligament

Medial meniscus

Posterior cruciate ligament

Medial condyle of tibia

Lateral condyle of tibia

Popliteus m.

Soleus m.

Posterior tibial a.

Posterior tibial v.

Posterior tibial v.

Posterior tibial a.

Biceps femoris m.

Lateral head of gastrocnemius m.

Biceps femoris tendon

Lateral condyle of femur

Articular cartilage

Articular capsule

Knee joint cavity

Lateral meniscus

Lateral intercondylar tubercle

Fibular collateral ligament

Head of fibula

Peroneal a.

Peroneal v.

Section of the knee through the posterior cruciate ligament and the medial and lateral menisci.
Peroneal and anterior and posterior tibial vessel are included in the lower portion of the section.

Coronal Section

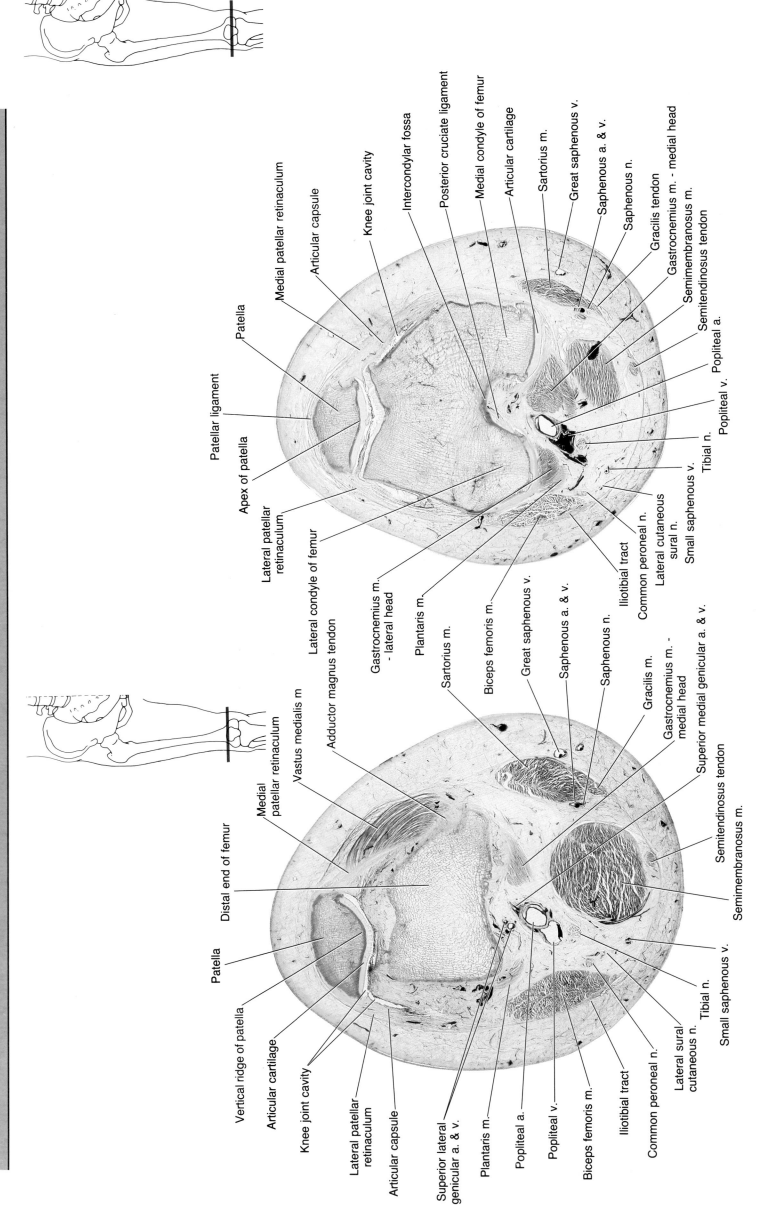

Medial patellar retinaculum

Articular capsule

Knee joint cavity

Intercondylar fossa

Posterior cruciate ligament

Medial condyle of femur

Articular cartilage

Sartorius m.

Great saphenous v.

Saphenous a. & v.

Saphenous n.

Gracilis tendon

Gastrocnemius m. - medial head

Semimembranosus m.

Semitendinosus tendon

Popliteal a.

Popliteal v.

Tibial n.

Small saphenous v.

Lateral cutaneous sural n.

Common peroneal n.

Iliotibial tract

Saphenous n.

Saphenous a. & v.

Great saphenous v.

Biceps femoris m.

Sartorius m.

Plantaris m.

Gastrocnemius m. - lateral head

Lateral condyle of femur

Adductor magnus tendon

Vastus medialis m

Medial patellar retinaculum

Lateral patellar retinaculum

Apex of patella

Patellar ligament

Patella

Distal end of femur

Patella

Vertical ridge of patella

Articular cartilage

Knee joint cavity

Articular capsule

Superior lateral genicular a. & v.

Plantaris m.

Popliteal a.

Popliteal v.

Biceps femoris m.

Iliotibial tract

Common peroneal n.

Lateral sural cutaneous n.

Tibial n.

Small saphenous v.

Semimembranosus m.

Semitendinosus tendon

Superior medial genicular a. & v.

Gastrocnemius m. - medial head

Gracilis m.

Saphenous n.

Saphenous a. & v.

Great saphenous v.

LOWER EXTREMITY.
Plate 7-11
Tranverse Section

LOWER EXTREMITY.
Plate 7-12
Transverse Section

Plate 7-11: Section of the knee through the patella and distal end of the femur proximal to the condyles.
Plate 7-12: Section of the knee through the patella and distal femur at the proximal end of the condyles.

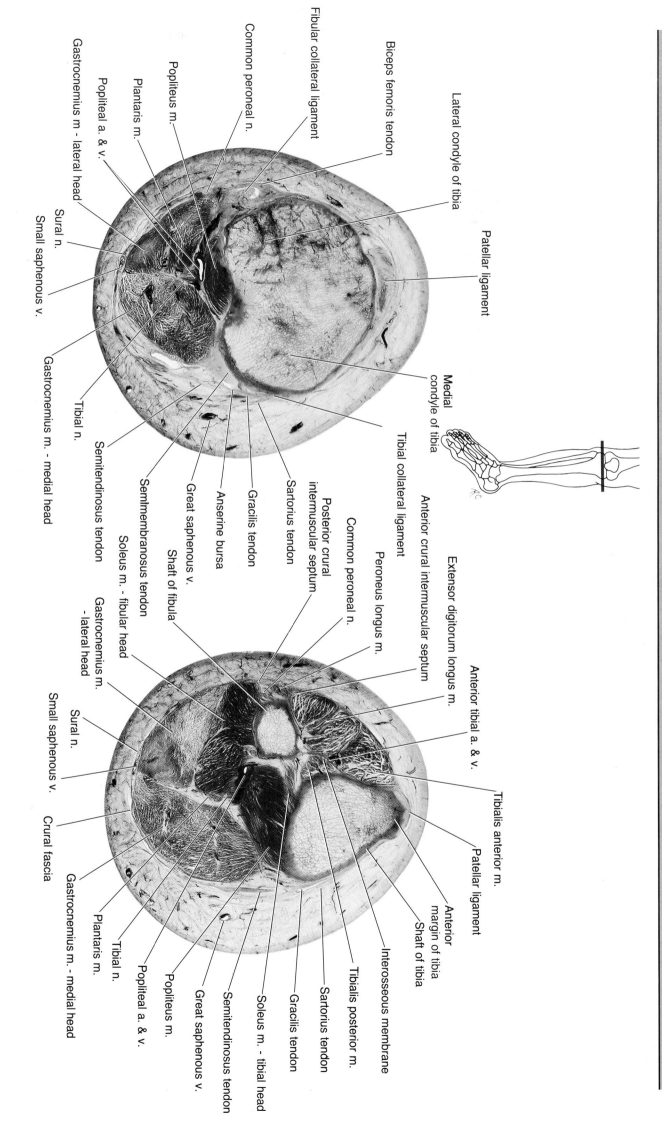

Plate 7-13: Section of the leg through the medial and lateral condyles of the tibia.
Plate 7-14: Section of the leg at the tibial tuberosity, including the insertion of the Popliteus on the tibia.

Lateral condyle of tibia

Biceps femoris tendon

Fibular collateral ligament

Common peroneal n.

Popliteus m.

Plantaris m.

Popliteal a. & v.

Gastrocnemius m - lateral head

Sural n.

Small saphenous v.

Gastrocnemius m. - medial head

Tibial n.

Semitendinosus tendon

Semimembranosus tendon

Great saphenous v.

Anserine bursa

Gracilis tendon

Sartorius tendon

Posterior crural intermuscular septum

Common peroneal n.

Peroneus longus m.

Tibial collateral ligament

Anterior crural intermuscular septum

Extensor digitorum longus m.

Patellar ligament

Medial condyle of tibia

Patellar ligament

Anterior tibial a. & v.

Tibialis anterior m.

Anterior margin of tibia

Shaft of tibia

Interosseous membrane

Tibialis posterior m.

Sartorius tendon

Gracilis tendon

Soleus m. - tibial head

Semitendinosus tendon

Great saphenous v.

Popliteus m.

Popliteal a. & v.

Tibial n.

Plantaris m.

Gastrocnemius m. - medial head

Crural fascia

Small saphenous v.

Sural n.

Gastrocnemius m. - lateral head

Soleus m. - fibular head

Gastrocnemius m. - lateral head

Shaft of fibula

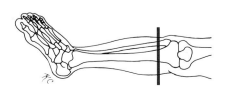

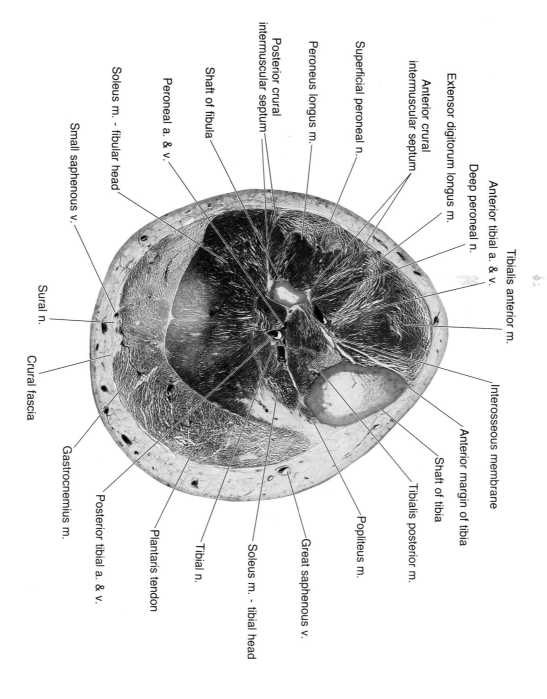

Tibialis anterior m.

Anterior tibial a. & v.

Deep peroneal n.

Extensor digitorum longus m.

Anterior crural
intermuscular septum

Peroneus longus m.

Superficial peroneal n.

Shaft of fibula

Posterior crural
intermuscular septum

Peroneal a. & v.

Soleus m. - fibular head

Small saphenous v.

Sural n.

Crural fascia

Gastrocnemius m.

Posterior tibial a. & v.

Plantaris tendon

Tibial n.

Soleus m. - tibial head

Great saphenous v.

Popliteus m.

Tibialis posterior m.

Shaft of tibia

Anterior margin of tibia

Interosseous membrane

LOWER EXTREMITY.
Plate 7-15

Section of the promimal leg through the bellies of the Gastrocnemius and Soleus muscles.

Transverse Section

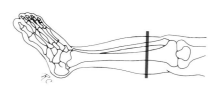

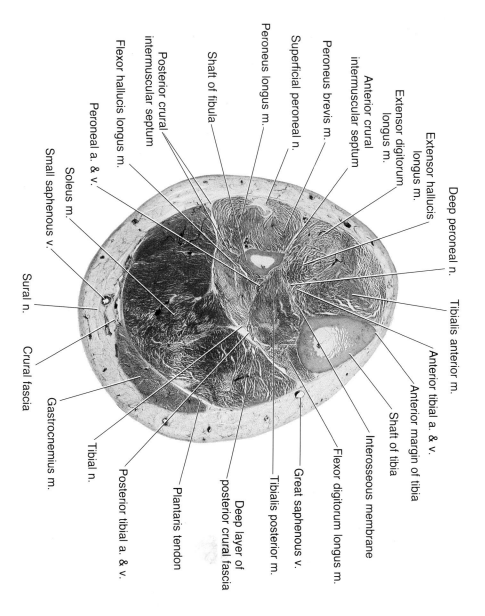

Deep peroneal n.

Extensor hallucis
longus m.

Extensor digitorum
longus m.

Anterior crural
intermuscular septum

Peroneus brevis m.

Superficial peroneal n.

Peroneus longus m.

Shaft of fibula

Posterior crural
intermuscular septum

Flexor hallucis longus m.

Peroneal a. & v.

Small saphenous v.

Soleus m.

Sural n.

Crural fascia

Gastrocnemius m.

Tibial n.

Posterior tibial a. & v.

Plantaris tendon

Deep layer of
posterior crural fascia

Tibialis posterior m.

Great saphenous v.

Flexor digitorum longus m.

Interosseous membrane

Shaft of tibia

Anterior margin of tibia

Anterior tibial a. & v.

Tibialis anterior m.

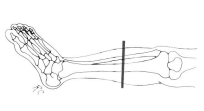

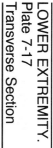

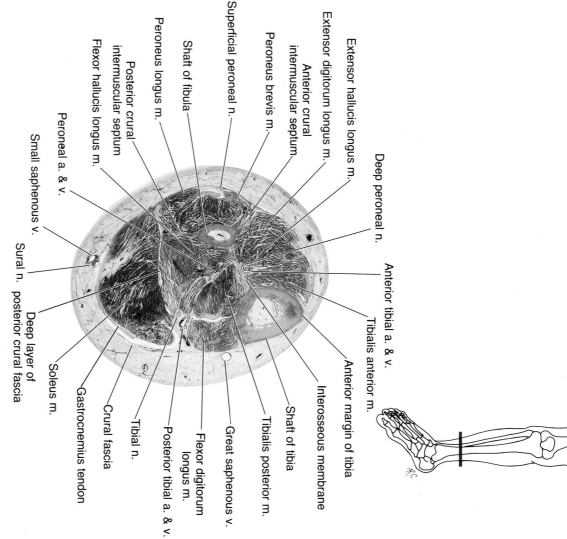

Deep peroneal n.

Extensor hallucis longus m.

Extensor digitorum longus m.

Anterior crural
intermuscular septum

Peroneus brevis m.

Superficial peroneal n.

Peroneus longus m.

Shaft of fibula

Posterior crural
intermuscular septum

Flexor hallucis longus m.

Peroneal a. & v.

Small saphenous v.

Sural n.

Anterior tibial a. & v.

Tibialis anterior m.

Anterior margin of tibia

Interosseous membrane

Shaft of tibia

Tibialis posterior m.

Great saphenous v.

Flexor digitorum
longus m.

Posterior tibial a. & v.

Tibial n.

Crural fascia

Gastrocnemius tendon

Deep layer of
posterior crural fascia

Soleus m.

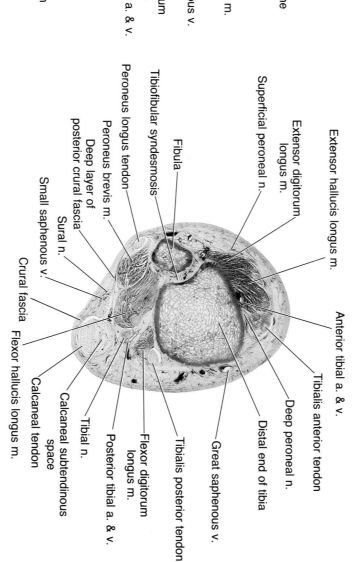

Peroneus longus tendon

Tibiofibular syndesmosis

Fibula

Peroneus brevis m.

Deep layer of
posterior crural fascia

Sural n.

Small saphenous v.

Crural fascia

Extensor hallucis longus m.

Extensor digitorum
longus m.

Superficial peroneal n.

Anterior tibial a. & v.

Tibialis anterior tendon

Deep peroneal n.

Distal end of tibia

Great saphenous v.

Tibialis posterior tendon

Flexor digitorum
longus m.

Posterior tibial a. & v.

Tibial n.

Calcaneal subtendinous
space

Calcaneal tendon

Flexor hallucis longus m.

LOWER EXTREMITY.
Plate 7-17
Transverse Section

Plate 7-17: Section of the mid-leg through the proximal end of the calcaneal tendon.
Plate 7-18: Section of the distal leg at tibia's fibular notch containing the interosseous tibiofibular ligament.

LOWER EXTREMITY.
Plate 7-18
Transverse Section

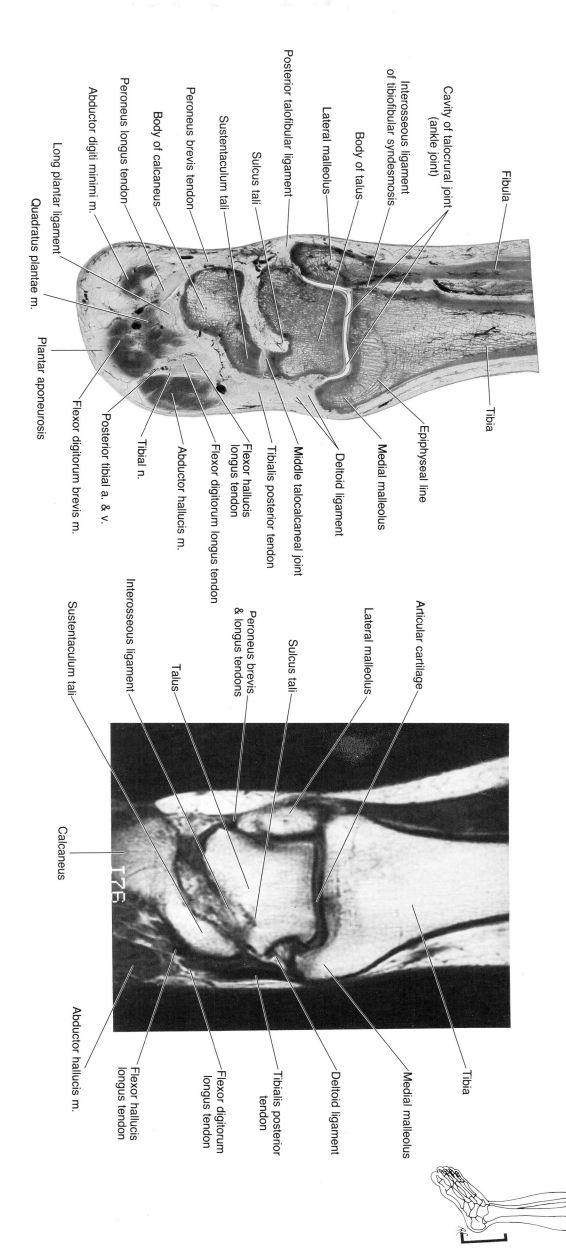

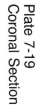

Fibula

Cavity of talocrural joint (ankle joint)

Interosseous ligament of tibiofibular syndesmosis

Body of talus

Lateral malleolus

Posterior talofibular ligament

Sulcus tali

Sustentaculum tali

Peroneus brevis tendon

Body of calcaneus

Peroneus longus tendon

Abductor digiti minimi m.

Long plantar ligament

Quadratus plantae m.

Plantar aponeurosis

Flexor digitorum brevis m.

Posterior tibial a. & v.

Tibial n.

Abductor hallucis m.

Flexor digitorum longus tendon

Flexor hallucis longus tendon

Tibialis posterior tendon

Middle talocalcaneal joint

Deltoid ligament

Medial malleolus

Epiphyseal line

Tibia

Articular cartilage

Lateral malleolus

Sulcus tali

Peroneus brevis & longus tendons

Talus

Interosseous ligament

Sustentaculum tali

Calcaneus

Abductor hallucis m.

Flexor hallucis longus tendon

Flexor digitorum longus tendon

Tibialis posterior tendon

Deltoid ligament

Medial malleolus

Tibia

Plate 7-19
Coronal Section

Plate 7-19
Coronal Section

Plate 7-19 MRI
Coronal Section

Sections of the ankle through the medial and lateral malleoli, talus, and calcaneus (including the sustentaculum tali). Portions of the distal tibiofibular, talocrural, and talocalcaneal joints are included.

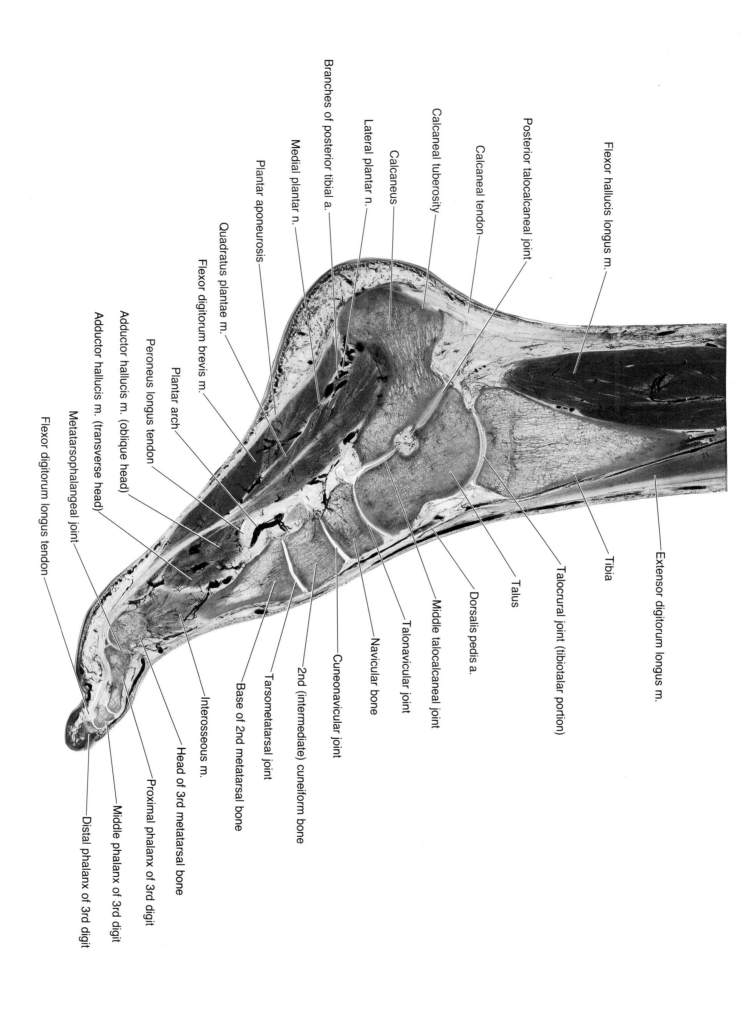

Flexor hallucis longus m.

Posterior talocalcaneal joint

Calcaneal tendon

Calcaneal tuberosity

Calcaneus

Lateral plantar n.

Branches of posterior tibial a.

Medial plantar n.

Plantar aponeurosis

Quadratus plantae m.

Flexor digitorum brevis m.

Plantar arch

Peroneus longus tendon

Adductor hallucis m. (oblique head)

Adductor hallucis m. (transverse head)

Metatarsophalangeal joint

Flexor digitorum longus tendon

Distal phalanx of 3rd digit

Middle phalanx of 3rd digit

Proximal phalanx of 3rd digit

Head of 3rd metatarsal bone

Interosseous m.

Base of 2nd metatarsal bone

Tarsometatarsal joint

2nd (intermediate) cuneiform bone

Cuneonavicular joint

Navicular bone

Talonavicular joint

Middle talocalcaneal joint

Dorsalis pedis a.

Talus

Talocrural joint (tibiotalar portion)

Tibia

Extensor digitorum longus m.

Slightly oblique section of the foot through the calcaneus, talus, navicular bone, 2nd cuneiform bone, 2nd metatarsal bone and phalanges of the third digit. The longitudinal arch of the foot is included.

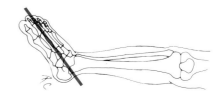

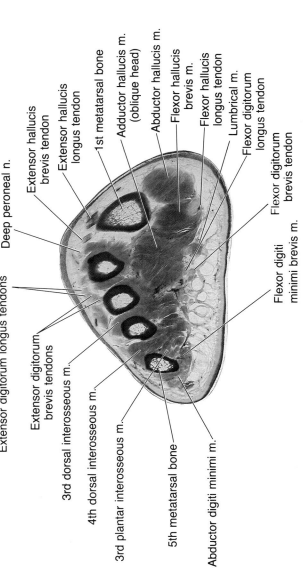

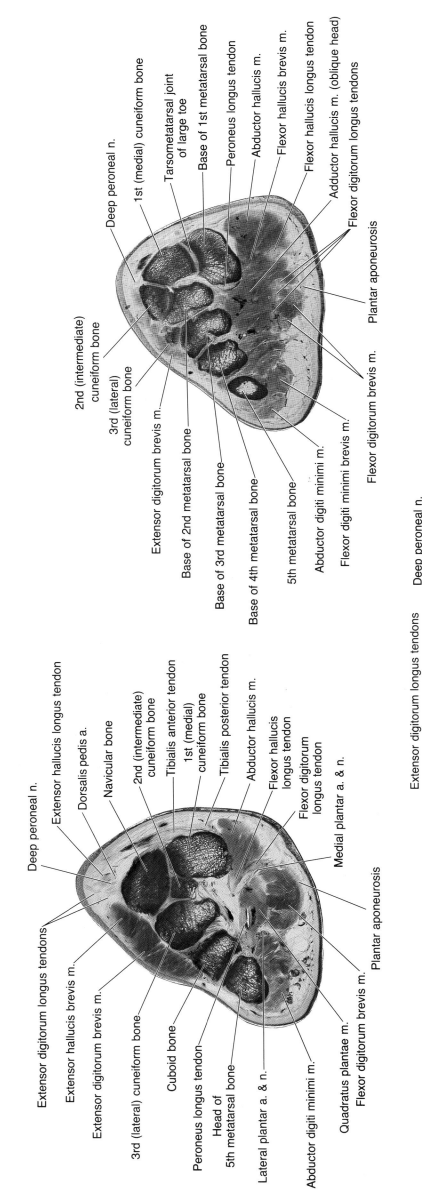

Deep peroneal n.

1st (medial) cuneiform bone
Tarsometatarsal joint of large toe
Base of 1st metatarsal bone
Peroneus longus tendon
Abductor hallucis m.
Flexor hallucis brevis m.
Flexor hallucis longus tendon
Adductor hallucis m. (oblique head)
Flexor digitorum longus tendons
Plantar aponeurosis

2nd (intermediate) cuneiform bone
3rd (lateral) cuneiform bone
Extensor digitorum brevis m.
Base of 2nd metatarsal bone
Base of 3rd metatarsal bone
Base of 4th metatarsal bone
5th metatarsal bone
Abductor digiti minimi m.
Flexor digiti minimi brevis m.
Flexor digitorum brevis m.

Deep peroneal n.
Extensor hallucis brevis tendon
Extensor hallucis longus tendon
1st metatarsal bone
Adductor hallucis m. (oblique head)
Abductor hallucis m.
Flexor hallucis brevis m.
Flexor hallucis longus tendon
Lumbrical m.
Flexor digitorum longus tendon
Flexor digitorum brevis tendon
Flexor digiti minimi brevis m.
Abductor digiti minimi m.
5th metatarsal bone
3rd plantar interosseous m.
4th dorsal interosseous m.
3rd dorsal interosseous m.
Extensor digitorum brevis tendons
Extensor digitorum longus tendons

Deep peroneal n.
Extensor digitorum longus tendons
Extensor hallucis longus tendon
Dorsalis pedis a.
Navicular bone
2nd (intermediate) cuneiform bone
Tibialis anterior tendon
1st (medial) cuneiform bone
Tibialis posterior tendon
Abductor hallucis m.
Flexor hallucis longus tendon
Flexor digitorum longus tendon
Medial plantar a. & n.
Plantar aponeurosis

Extensor hallucis brevis m.
Extensor digitorum brevis m.
3rd (lateral) cuneiform bone
Cuboid bone
Peroneus longus tendon
Head of 5th metatarsal bone
Lateral plantar a. & n.
Abductor digiti minimi m.
Quadratus plantae m.
Flexor digitorum brevis m.

Tranverse Section

Series of sections of the foot through the navicular and cuneiform bones (Plate 7-21), the cuneiform bones and the head of the metatarsal bones (Plate 7-22), and the metatarsal bones (Plate 7-23).

INDEX

144

gluteus maximus, 82, 83, 101-111,115-120, 122-127
gluteus medius, 83, 101-107, 109, 115-117, 122-124
gluteus minimus, 83, 101-106, 115-117, 122-124
gracilis, 111, 120, 125-129, 134, 135
hyoglossus, 4, 25-28
iliacus, 83, 101-103, 122-124
iliocostalis, 83
iliocostalis lumborum, 84-89, 91, 93-98
iliopsoas, 83, 104-109, 115-119, 122, 123, 125
infraspinatus, 37-40, 61, 65, 67-70
intercostal, 37-39, 61, 64, 65, 67, 68
    external, 69-71, 73, 75, 77-79, 84-86
    innermost, 69, 71, 75, 78, 84-86
    internal, 69-71, 73, 75, 77-79, 84-86
interosseous, of foot, 140
    of hand, dorsal, 55, 56
        palmar, 55, 56
ischiocavernosus, 110, 111
latissimus dorsi, 41, 61, 71, 73, 75, 77-79, 83-89, 91, 93-96
levator anguli oris, 21, 22, 24
levator ani, 82, 106-111, 114, 117-119
levator labii superioris, 19-21
levator labii superioris alaeque nasi, 15-17, 19
levator palpebrae, 3, 4, 11
levator scapulae, 28-34, 38, 62-65
levator veli palatini, 5, 22
longissimus capitis, 24-26, 28-31
longissimus cervicis, 29-32
longissimus thoracis, 82, 84-89, 91, 93-98
longus capitis, 5, 21-24, 26, 28-32
longus colli, 5, 23, 24, 26, 28-32, 63
limbrical, of foot, 141
    of hand, 55, 57
masseter, 3-5, 19-26
mentalis, 26, 28
multifidus, 30-34, 84, 85, 94-98
mylohyoid, 2-4, 26-29
nasalis, 15-17, 19
oblique, inferior, 3, 15, 16
    superior, 3, 4, 11
obliquus capitis inferior, 25, 26
obliquus capitis superior, 24, 25
obturator externus, 82, 83, 107-110, 116-119, 122-124
obturator internus, 82, 83, 103-109, 116-118, 122-124
occipitofrontalis, 13-15
omohyoid, 32-34, 37, 62-64
opponens digiti minimi, 55, 57
opponens pollicis, 54, 55
orbicularis oculi, 13-16, 19
orbicularis oris, 22, 23, 25, 27
palatoglossus, 25
palatopharyngeus, 23, 25, 26, 28, 29
palmar interosseous, hand, 55
palmaris brevis, 54, 55
palmaris longus, 49-53
pectineus, 82, 104-110, 116-119, 122, 123, 125
pectoralis major, 38-41, 61, 64-71, 73, 75, 77-79, 83
pectoralis minor, 38-41, 61, 65-71
peroneus, brevis, 137-139
    longus, 135-141
pharyngeal constrictor, 23, 24
    inferior, 5, 28-34
    middle, 5, 26, 28, 30
    superior, 25, 26
piriformis, 82, 83, 102, 103, 105, 115, 123, 124
plantaris, 131, 134-137
platysma, 2, 4, 26, 28-34, 62, 63
popliteus, 130-133, 135, 136
pronator quadratus, 53, 54, 56
pronator teres, 45-47, 49, 50
    ulnar head, 47
psoas major, 82, 93-98, 101-103
pterygoid, lateral, 5, 19-21, 22
    medial, 5, 21-26
pyramidalis, 105-107
quadratus femoris, 83, 108-110, 116-119, 124
quadratus lumborum, 83, 94-98, 124
quadratus plantae, 139-141
rectus abdominis, 60, 61, 82, 83, 87-89, 91, 93-98, 100-103, 105,

    114, 115, 124
    tendinous intersection, 61, 83
rectus capitis anterior, 22, 24
rectus capitis lateralis, 24
rectus femoris, 104-110, 116-120, 125-129
rectus, inferior, 4, 15, 16
    lateral, 4, 12-14
    medial, 3, 4, 13, 14
    superior, 4, 11
rhomboid major, 38-41, 62-65, 67-71
rhomboid minor, 33, 34, 38, 39, 62-65, 67
sacrospinalis, 64, 67, 68, 70, 71, 75, 79
sartorius, 102-110, 115-120, 125-129, 134, 135
scalenus, anterior, 30, 32-34, 62-64
    medius, 29-34, 62, 63
    posterior, 30-34, 62, 63
senimembranosus, 120, 125-129, 132, 134, 135
semispinalis, capitis, 24-26, 28-34
    cervicis, 28-34
semitendinosus, 83, 120, 124-129, 134, 135
serratus, anterior, 37-41, 61, 63-65, 67-71, 73, 75, 77-79, 84-87,
    posterior, inferior, 88, 89, 91, 94
        superior, 34
soleus, 131-133, 135-138
    fibular head, 135, 136
    tibial head, 135, 136
spinalis cervicis, 31-34
splenius, capitis, 24-26, 28-34, 62, 63
    cervicis, 62, 63
sternocleidomastoid, 24-26, 28-34, 60, 62-64
sternohyoid, 2, 30-34, 62-65, 67
sternothyroid, 2, 32-34, 62-65, 67
styloglossus, 25, 26
stylohyoid, 26, 28
stylopharyngeus, 23, 25, 26
subclavius, 61, 64
subscapularis, 36-41, 61, 65, 67-71
supinator, 48-51
supraspinatus, 36-38, 61, 64, 65
temporalis, 4, 5, 10, 11, 13-16, 19-22
tensor fasciae latae, 102-110, 115-120, 123, 125, 126
tensor veli palatini, 21, 22
teres major, 37, 40, 41, 69-71
teres minor, 37-41, 61, 65, 67-71
thenar, 55
thyroarytenoid, 32
thyrohyoid, 5, 30, 31
tibialis, anterior, 131, 135-138, 141
    posterior, 131, 135-139, 141
transversospinal, 63, 64, 67, 68, 70, 71, 75, 79
transversus, abdominis, 91, 93-98, 101, 102
    thoracis, 75, 77, 78
trapezius, 25, 26, 28-34, 37-40, 61-65, 67-71, 73, 75, 77-79, 82
triceps, brachii, 43-45, 48
    lateral head, 37, 40-42, 69-71
    long head, 40-42, 68-71
urogenital diaphragm, 100
vastus intermedius, 110, 118-120, 125-129, 131
vastus lateralis, 107-110, 118-120, 122, 123, 125-129, 131
vastus medialis, 120, 123, 125-129, 132, 134
zygomaticus major, 21, 22, 24

Musculi pectinati, 77

Nasal bone, 2, 12, 13, 60
Nasal cavity, 2-4, 12-21
Nasal meatus
    inferior, 3, 21
    middle, 3
Nasal spetum, 18
Nasopharynx, 2, 5
Navicular bone, 140, 141
Nerve
    alveolar, inferior, 3, 4, 22, 24-26
    axillary, 37
    common palmar digital, 57
    common peroneal, 129
    cranial
        abducens, 19, 20